Talking Points

Talking Points
Second Edition

Pamela J. Maraldo, PhD, RN, FAAN
Peter Preziosi, EdM, RN
Leah F. Binder

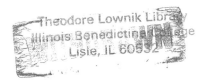
Pub. No. 41-2287

National League for Nursing Press • New York

Copyright © 1991 by
National League for Nursing Press

ISBN 0-88737-449-2

This book was edited by Rachel Schaperow and designed by Allan
Graubard. Publications Development Company was the typesetter and
Northeastern Press was the printer and binder. The cover was designed by
Lillian Welsh.

Manufactured in the United States of America

About the Authors

Pamela J. Maraldo, PhD, RN, FAAN, has served as Executive Director of the National League for Nursing, a coalition of individual and agency members that promotes quality nursing care to the public, since 1983. During this time, she has led a programmatic and financial revitalization of the organization. Prior to assuming this post, she established and administered the NLN Office of Public Affairs, which has become an authoritative source on health policy issues and a frequent contributor to legislative and regulatory formulation on Capitol Hill. In this capacity, she initiated health policy dialogue with the White House and Congress and has played an advocacy role in encouraging active nursing participation in the political arena on the national, state, and local levels.

Peter Preziosi, EdM, RN, is Director of Public Policy for the National League for Nursing. He was formerly Special Assistant to the Senior Vice President for Marketing and Development at NLN and has been employed in nursing positions at Memorial Sloan-Kettering Cancer Center, Bellevue Hospital Center, and New York Hospital-Cornell Medical Center. He is presently completing a dual PhD/MGA degree at the University of Pennsylvania in the School of Nursing and the Fels Center of Government.

Leah F. Binder is a writer from Portland, Maine, and was formerly Special Assistant to the Executive Director of NLN. She has a bachelor's degree in Politics from Brandeis University.

Preface

Talking Points was developed with an eye toward creating an easy-to-use reference tool for people interested in nursing and health care issues. Since we believe communication skills are most essential, we begin with a section on working with the media and legislators.

The question and answer section is divided into the major categories of cost, access, and quality—very similar to the way policymakers analyze the current health care system. The questions selected were based on the requests NLN most frequently receives for information regarding nursing and health care issues. The question-and-answer format provides the reader with quick access to the information.

The resource list includes an annotated bibliography and lists of health policy journals, newsletters, and nursing organizations.

We hope that the readers of *Talking Points* will use this tool to promote nurses' views on nursing and health care.

Contents

Introduction

Nurses have a unique and extremely valuable perspective on the challenges and possibilities we face in our nation's health care delivery system. Too often, however, the nursing perspective is not represented in the nation's policy dialogue. As a result, policymakers and the public remain unaware of nursing solutions to some of our most pressing health care dilemmas. Yet many crisis issues in health care today require nursing expertise to solve; the most daunting challenges point to nurses as the providers and experts of choice.

As the nation's health care price tag escalates precariously, nurses offer proven methods for lowering costs; as the nursing shortage rages, nurses demonstrate how to solve it; as the incidence of chronic illness grows, nurses offer expertise on providing cost-effective, compassionate care; as the percentage of elderly in the population increases, nurses provide effective health solutions to the special needs of graying Americans.

It is thus critical to the future of health care that nurses translate the nursing experience and vision into a concrete public voice. *Talking Points* is an effort to give nurses—faculty, students, and nurses in practice—some assistance in addressing the media and talking about key nursing issues in class or with colleagues. But *Talking Points* is even more than answers to the most commonly asked questions about nurses and nursing. *Talking Points* shows you how to communicate with the broadcast as well as print media, legislators, and other leaders who influence public opinion. Nurses must shape the perceptions of these media influentials regarding nursing and health care so they will become knowledgeable about nursing and support constructive change.

Managing the Media

The power of the media to shape public opinion and, ultimately, change behavior is well-known. The fate of many an emerging cause or rising luminary has been sealed before tens of millions during a few seconds of national network exposure.

Such is the awe in which the media are held that individuals and groups seeking to promote or influence often race, unprepared, to bask in the media's magical rays. In fact, there are limitations to what can be accomplished through the media, and there are hazards to be avoided. Media relations is both an art—requiring good interpersonal skills, sound judgment, reliable instincts, and quick wits—as well as a science with established principles and protocols.

Media relations means far more than seeking publicity for an isolated event. It represents a long-term partnership that should be undertaken with a sense of commitment and perseverance. One news item stating one opinion from the nursing perspective is only a first step in building a voice for nursing in the media. By establishing a relationship with the media, you become an ongoing conduit of information from your profession to the public while also providing a vital public service.

Media relations cannot be relied on as the sole strategy in a campaign to shape public opinion. Along with other public relations activities designed to reach target groups of influentials, and with political action, it should be part of a total marketing plan.

Nor can media relations be used to "create" a new reality. It can alter public perception and foster consumer demand. This will only backfire, however, if the day-to-day experiences of the consumer public differ from expectations that have been cultivated through the media.

Resolving the question of whether to enter the media arena involves strategic planning and positioning. It is important to define your objectives—and then assess strengths and weaknesses—to determine the appropriateness of the objectives and your ability to follow through on selected opportunities.

Marketing nursing care successfully in a rapidly changing and competitive health care delivery system requires the strategic use of mass communications to reach the largest numbers of consumers, providers, and policymakers. Become successful by harnessing the activities of nursing and health care organizations to accent the message you want to get across to the public. Understand the goals of their public relations departments and coordinate activities for a more solid, effective, and strong approach that hits hard across the media.

Careful planning is essential. Define and research your message. Determine which kind of media will offer the most appropriate vehicle to successfully communicate your perspective. The community newspaper or local radio station is worlds apart from *The Today Show* or *The Washington Post*.

Consider the legislative, regulatory, economic, and environmental factors likely to influence the public's receptivity to your message. Creating a public ground swell hinges on linking your message to the current public agenda. Competing with other developments or events for media attention may influence the way you ultimately package your message. Know what the public's agenda is and interweave it into your message. The only way people will stand up and take notice of what you are saying is if the message seems relevant to the times. Don't forget to be prepared with responses to the public's reactions if your message happens to be controversial.

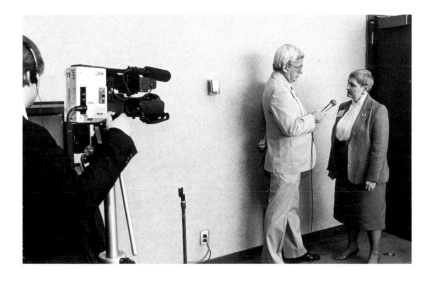

Working Effectively
with the Media

As a first step, let media representatives know who you are and what types of data, expert commentary, and contacts you can provide. Make sure to stress whenever possible that you are there to assist them (whether or not a particular story they are working on will result in direct coverage for you or your organization).

Rare indeed are the opportunities for presenting an opinion or fact as an isolated nugget of wisdom. Even publicists for the U.S. President refine White House news to give the media an "angle" for the story—establishing timeliness and connection with issues of import to the public. Thus, for example, the least effective means of attracting press attention to the value of primary nursing care is to write a press release proclaiming that viewpoint and stating supportive statistics. Instead, relate the facts to an angle. Announce the one-year anniversary of a local nursing center; announce the results of a study where nurses lowered health care costs; relate the need for primary nursing care to recently released statistics on the increasing rate of infant mortality in your community.

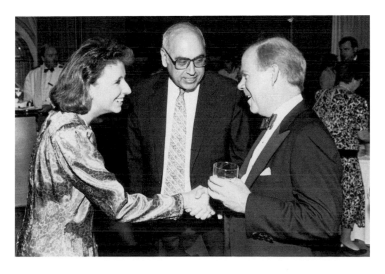

An instant angle often emerges from major and minor holidays, which can be tied to an issue. Birthdays of famous people or community leaders are often opportunities to honor role models and reflect on philosophical or political beliefs and goals.

Once you are recognized as a timely source of accurate information, the media will be more likely to contact you about nursing and health care stories and be more responsive to your press releases, feature and talk show suggestions, and public service announcements. Your relationship with the media will proceed much more smoothly if they perceive you as a partner in the process of bringing the news to the public and a valuable source of expertise in helping them develop stories, rather than as a single-purpose publicity seeker.

Be sensitive to the particular needs of the medium you are working with at any given time, and tailor your approach accordingly. What you believe to be news may not be considered as such by the press. In that case, respect their judgment and try to learn from the experience. When planning events and activities, ask yourself what would make for interesting coverage. You can't sell the media an empty bill of goods, but if you have a story to tell, there's nothing wrong with shaping it to fit their needs.

Candor and honesty are essential in dealing with the media. If you once pitch a reporter a story that isn't solid, that reporter will never trust your judgment again. If your don't know how to answer a question, say so—you're not expected to know everything. Find the answer and get back to the reporter. Remember that deadlines rule. Always find out what deadline a reporter must meet and provide needed information within that time frame.

If you have reason to suspect that an unfavorable story is in the making, don't refuse to speak to the reporter involved or use the guilt-by-avoidance "no comment." If you are honest and convincing enough, you may be able to turn the story around. Don't demand to review press copy before the story runs; this will only antagonize the writer. Never babble "off the record"; there's no such thing.

It's far more constructive in the long run to be proactive, rather than reactive, in negotiating the media maze. Don't harp on what you consider to be unfavorable press. There are always numerous viewpoints competing to mold a story, and your perspective is not going to come out on top every time. Instead of berating reporters or editors about an instance of bad press, concentrate your efforts on building credibility and trust so that they will ask your opinion next time.

Finally, remember that any media message must be repeated and reinforced over and over again through a variety of channels. We live in a media–intensive society in which only a fraction of messages register with any individual consumer, and all messages are quickly buried by the next round of media bombardment.

Preparing for the Interview

In many of the interview situations you will encounter, your message will not reach an audience directly. Your words will be filtered through the reporter's and editor's interpretations of that message. Especially in edited interviews, careful selection by the reporter may change the thrust of your interview. While you can control the outcome of an interview to a certain degree, it is the reporter's perceptions that will be reflected in the end product.

Your goal during an interview or media situation is to reach an audience with your story. You will accomplish this objective by leading or controlling the interview as much as possible.

It is particularly important that you fully understand the specific medium and situation; the interviewer; his or her objectives; the audience; and your own communications, objectives, and messages. The following guidelines should be used to prepare for—and capitalize on—any media interview situation.

Evaluate the Situation

■ *Subject.* Determine what the reporter/interviewer is looking for. Is it a story about the nursing shortage or a specific health policy issue?

■ *Medium/Publication's Focus.* Learn the focus or needs of the reporter's publication or station so that your answers will be relevant to that audience. What does the medium specialize in? What are the audience's main concerns?

■ *Format.* Determine the interview format. Is it print, radio, TV, or magazine? Is it a one-on-one interview, group interview, panel discussion, or listener/watcher call-in?

■ *Time.* Consider the length of the interview and the length of the edited product.

■ *Other Sources.* Ask the reporter if other information will be used, who will be contacted, and how your information will be used.

■ *Deadlines.* Every reporter has a deadline—ask the reporter what it is. If you are faced with difficult questions during the interview that are not within your area of expertise, don't feel obligated to answer on the spot.

The Press Release

Your basic tool for alerting the media to any event, development, or activity is the press release, which is best followed up with a telephone call or personal contact. Send the release to the news editor or city editor of a print publication, and to the news director or assignment editor of a radio or television station. Don't expect coverage from every release, but do keep sending them. This will keep your name and activities in the minds of media representatives and may result in future coverage. If the story is appropriate, don't neglect small local media, who will be the most inclined to use your material and to use more of it.

Keep in mind the following tips when planning your release:

■ Write simply and directly. Be specific.

■ Be brief. Keep your release to a page or two, if possible.

■ Date the release for the day it will arrive on the editor's desk.

■ Write objectively. Assign opinions to specific individuals. Use quotes to praise or criticize.

■ The release should lend itself to skimming. Paragraphs should not exceed two to three sentences. Snappy headings and subheadings can help.

■ Follow the golden editorial rule: answer the "Five W's" in the first paragraph. What happened, where and when, who is involved, and why it is important.

■ Legend has it that editors cut stories with scissors, lopping off paragraphs at the bottom of the story. So, when writing press releases, deal with the Five W's first, then follow with details and quotes in order of priority.

■ Don't belabor credentials. Editors and readers of a professional journal may be interested in a long list of professional achievements and honors; for the consumer press, an individual's affiliation and title are usually sufficient.

■ Follow standard format or your release won't make it far from the envelope. At the top of the release, type your organization's name, address, and telephone number; the date on which the item may be used; and the name and telephone number of a single contact person who can answer questions and provide further information. Type the release double- or triple-spaced, with fairly wide margins, on 8-1/2 × 11 paper, preferably on only one side of each sheet. Type "more" at the bottom of each page except the last, which should be marked "30" or "#" at the bottom.

■ The purpose of your group or organization may not be immediately clear to readers unfamiliar with your field. At the end of the release, include a brief description of your group's purpose.

Print Media

News treatment is only one option for print coverage. It is the area in which the competition is the greatest, and is, by nature, subject to late-breaking developments that can overshadow or supplant your story.

Features coverage is less timely and more in-depth, so don't forget to contact health, life-style, or other editors who may be interested in your message. A news editor who feels that your story has a features slant may also pass the release on to a features editor.

A photograph may not be worth the proverbial thousand words, but it ought to be considered. If you have an activity or display planned that would readily lend itself to photographic coverage, let the press know. Send a memo to the photo editor or add a brief note describing photographic opportunities at the end of the press release, and then follow up with a telephone call.

Radio

In addition to news treatment, the other major opportunities for radio coverage of your story are talk shows and public service announcements (PSAs).

Radio talk shows—which may be in a discussion format, a call-in format, or a combination of both—offer numerous opportunities to reach the public. Before you contact a talk show producer to suggest programs, do some basic homework so as not to waste the producer's time or yours. Be familiar with the format of the show and with the range of topics it covers. Provide specific suggestions for discussion, as well as for participants. Make sure the participants you suggest are the most articulate available—they may not necessarily be the highest ranking or the best known—and make sure that they are fully briefed and in command of all pertinent facts.

Although radio stations are no longer obligated to air PSAs to the extent they once were, many still use PSAs regularly. These announcements may recognize an event of interest to the community, promote a public service, or invite the public to attend an activity or meeting. Although it is preferable to provide the station with professional quality tapes, some stations may work from scripts you provide. Most PSAs are 10 or 20 seconds long.

Television

Many of the basic principles that apply to radio news, talk shows, and PSAs also apply here, but television is a medium unto itself. It is a "hot," immediate, emotional medium that brings the world into the living room and reaches countless people who do not read newspapers or magazines regularly. A few minutes of TV exposure will often produce a much more lasting impression than in-depth print coverage. Television is the most specialized medium, and it is the one in which it is the most difficult to obtain coverage. For TV news coverage, it is not enough that your story be timely and newsworthy—it must be visually effective as well.

Carefully choose your representatives for TV interviews and discussions. Many knowledgeable people who can effectively handle a print interview lack the poise, succinctness, and talent necessary for effective television communication. Even the accomplished public speaker may be surprised by the way the TV camera can distort or exaggerate body language. Seeing yourself on videotape can be an enlightening and educational experience, and professional media training is desirable for anyone who will be making a publicity tour. Remember that if a program is taped, much of the footage can be edited out. Just as you write a press release so that it can be readily cut by an editor, you must pace a television interview so that any given segment can achieve maximum impact.

The Press Conference

If you're thinking of holding a press conference, be certain that it will generate news of interest to reporters and their editors and, above all, make sure your message is timely. Members of the press must be given a time-sensitive "hook," or else they may not attend. Announce the press conference with a short, one-page press release, and always follow up with phone calls.

Plan the conference around the needs of the media you most want to attract (evening television news programs need their news in the morning, while morning newspapers need theirs in the afternoon or early evening). Put together press kits of relevant materials (fact sheets, issues "backgrounders," biographies and photographs of principal people, as well as press releases), and remember to send them to reporters who could not attend.

Rehearse spokespersons with likely questions, especially the tough ones. Check equipment, such as microphones, and make sure everything is in working order. Plan to have sufficient staff to manage traffic, "press flesh," and resolve the inevitable behind-the-scenes problems of any such undertaking.

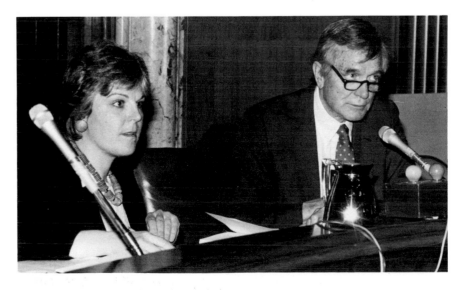

Communicating with Legislators

I f every nurse maintained steady correspondence with legislators, the nursing constituency would be far better represented by our government. Legislators pay close attention to constituent communications—a letter or call to your elected official is never wasted time.

Beyond writing letters or making phone calls, however, is the more complex process of strategizing politically to advance nursing's agenda in Congress. Nurses who undertake to organize politically must develop good working relationships with legislators and legislators' staff members. To get them to hear your message, you need to be well-prepared and articulate, know how the legislative process works, and understand at what specific points you can intervene.

First and most important, make sure you understand the legislative process. For information on the specific political structures of your city and state, plus directories of elected officials, contact your local Chamber of Commerce or League of Women Voters office. For information on the federal legislative process, consult standard American government texts, your local League of Women Voters (or the national office in Washington, DC), or *Key Concepts in Public Policy: Student Workbook* (NLN, 1986).

Whether you plan to speak out on an issue by visiting your legislator or presenting testimony, you must do some basic homework. First, learn all you can about the topic or piece of legislation. Contact the government relations staff of an organization likely to be involved (such as the American Nurses' Association or the National League for Nursing) to obtain available information. Find out how they are targeting their activities and how you can be kept up-to-date. This will help you avoid duplicated or wasted efforts.

Before contacting your elected representative, learn all you can about his or her political background: party affiliation, length of time in office, next time up for reelection, committee memberships, issues of particular concern. You can obtain this information from the legislator's local office, from a nurses' association, or from a nurses' political action committee (PAC). It's also a good idea to find out whether a nurses' PAC has endorsed the legislator in the past. Finally, and most important, find out what the legislator's stand has been on nursing and health care issues.

One last piece of information is crucial when you are promoting a specific bill or policy—its cost implications. How will the course of action you advocate save money, promote efficiency, or generate new revenues? How long will it take before an initial outlay is earned back in decreased costs? Legislators are reluctant to vote for new allocations these days without knowing the financial implications.

Writing Letters

Letter writing is one of the most effective and persuasive forms of lobbying because you, the voter, are taking the time to express your viewpoint. Letters should be directed to sympathetic as well as opposing legislators, because elected officials need proof of the presence of a committed constituency for every issue on which they take a side. To make your letter stand out among the thousands your legislator receives, follow these tips:

- *Identify Yourself.* Mention the state, congressional or legislative district, city or county in which you are a voter. Mention your professional affiliation, but use your own stationery, not agency stationery. A letter is better than a postcard or telegram. Sign your name, and use "RN" after it. Be sure your address is on the letter as well as on the envelope. Envelopes sometimes get thrown away before the letter is answered.

- *Be Specific.* When writing about legislation, use the bill number (H.R. 1490, S. 1402) or the title (Nursing Research Construction Act or Nurse Shortage Reduction Act) if your know them. If not, briefly describe the issue that concerns you.

- *Be Brief.* Write about one bill or issue at a time. Write on selected important issues not more than once or twice on each subject. Quality not quantity is what counts. A one-page letter will surely be read and is always the most effective.

- *Be Timely.* Timing is important. Try to write about a bill while it is in committee, not after a key vote has been taken. Your legislator will be more responsive to your appeal at that time rather than after the bill has been approved by a committee. Know what committees your legislator serves on and indicate in the letter if the bill is being brought before any of those committees.

- *Explain Your Position.* Briefly state why you are for or against the legislation. As a nurse, a taxpayer, or a consumer, say in your own words how the bill or amendment will affect you. Form letters are not as effective as original ones. Explain how the issue will affect you, your business, or your profession, or what effect it will have on your state or community. Don't forget that a bill can change as it moves through the legislative process. Urge your legislator to oppose crippling amendments or support strengthening ones.

- *Ask for a Response.* Urge your legislator to take action—support or oppose a bill, co-sponsor an amendment, or whatever action you would like taken. Request a reply to your letter. Remember to keep copies of all correspondence for your files. This information will be helpful to the lobbying efforts of your local, state, or national professional association.

- *Be Polite.* Don't be threatening, demanding, or abusive. That's an immediate turn-off. Express your appreciation for work well done, a good speech, favorable vote, or fine leadership in committee or on the floor.

- *Address it Properly.* For Congress:

U.S. Senator	U.S. Representative
Honorable Jane Doe	Honorable John Doe
United States Senate	House of Representatives
Washington, DC 20510	Washington, DC 20515
Dear Senator Doe:	Dear Representative Doe:

Write to senators, delegates, or assembly members in care of their state capitols.

Write to local officials in care of their city, town, or county government addresses. These can be found in your phone book.

- *Write it and Mail it.* Once you've taken the time to write a letter, using these suggestions or adopting a style of your own, don't forget to *mail it right away.* Remember, the timeliness of your communication is as important as what you've written.

Meeting with Your Legislator

Politicians are just people, and the unwritten rules for lobbying and political influence are the same as those for other social situations. You must develop a relationship with the legislator or staff member, get to know her or him and let her or him get to know you, before you ask for what you want. It will be easier for you to establish an effective relationship if you keep in mind the following tips:

■ Call ahead to make an appointment, asking to meet with the legislator. If the member is not available, ask to meet with the staff person who handles health issues. The staff person is a major influence in your representative's decision making.

■ Prepare in advance. Know your legislator's background and the history of the legislation you're discussing.

■ Dress conservatively in business attire. First impressions are important.

■ Introduce yourself at the beginning of the visit and state what you want to discuss, referring to specific issues or bills.

■ Ask the legislator what her or his position is on the issues or bills.

■ Be prepared to explain, in basic terms, nursing practice and nurses' legislative concerns. Many legislators and staff members are unfamiliar with the nursing profession. If possible, be prepared with facts about nursing practice in your state or district.

■ Ask if the legislator has heard others' opinions about this issue or bill. Ask what the supporters are saying; ask who the opponents are and what their arguments are.

■ Provide written information—a fact sheet or summary of your position, no longer than one page, to leave with the legislator.

- Offer to provide additional information if you don't have data at hand, but don't make promises you can't keep.

- Follow up with a thank-you note and express your thoughts about the visit.

- Keep a written record of the visit for your files; notify government liaison staff at professional nursing organizations so that they can follow up.

- Spend time with your legislators even if their positions are not in agreement with yours. You can lessen the intensity of their positions and maintain contact for subsequent issues.

- Ask what type of support the legislator would like in bills she or he is sponsoring in Congress. Quid pro quos are important in politics.

Preparing and Presenting Testimony

Presenting testimony at a legislative hearing is like producing a play. You must write a script (the testimony), select actors (the witnesses), and allow for rehearsal time (briefings). Legislative hearings are opportunities for interested parties to speak directly to legislators in a formal, well–publicized setting.

Keeping informed about hearings is the first step to presenting testimony. Have your name placed on the mailing lists of committees that are responsible for nursing and health care issues, or write to the committee chairperson to request the date of the hearing on a specific bill. In writing and presenting testimony, follow these tips:

- Become familiar with the jurisdiction of legislative committees, their subcommittees, and their membership.

- Identify bills that would have the most impact in areas of concern to you. Consult other professional nursing organizations to coordinate your efforts and energies.

- Write the chairperson of the subcommittee or committee that will hold the hearing and ask to be notified of the date. Find out the ground rules: time limitations, length of testimony, number of copies of printed testimony needed, deadline for submitting advance copies of testimony.

- Do not request the opportunity to present oral testimony on bills of marginal interest or to present oral testimony if a written statement inserted in the printed hearing record would suffice.

- Prepare testimony, in accordance with the ground rules, that agrees with approved policies of your parent organization.

- Select a witness knowledgeable in the subject area who will abide by the time limitations, preferably one who is from the chairperson's state or district.

- Notify elected representatives of your appearance, especially if they serve on the committee or subcommittee holding the hearing.

- Do not guess at the answer to a question. Instead, ask to submit the requested information at a later date.

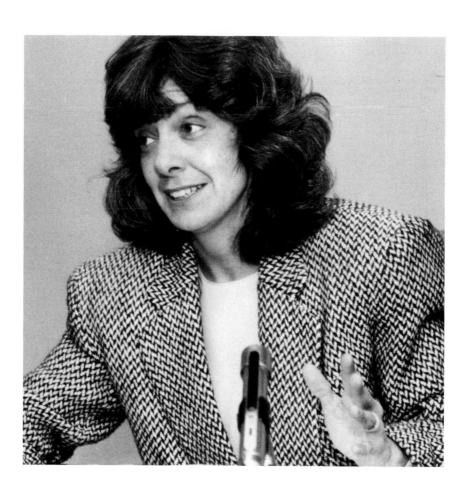

Questions and Answers About Nursing and Health Care

The rapidly changing health care marketplace concerns all individuals in our nation. Debates surface around three central themes: cost, access, and quality. We divided the wide spectrum of issues into key categories, using a question and answer format, to aid you in communicating with a reporter, legislator, colleague, or even your neighbor.

Health Costs: A National Crisis

Q *What is the greatest source of concern that the public has with the health care delivery system?*

A Costs. Nearly 12 percent of America's gross national product is spent on health care, a staggering $650 billion. That means the average American works 43 days a year to pay his or her share of the nation's health care price tag. Costs are soaring much faster than the rate of inflation.

In recent years the business community has also lent its considerable clout to the debate. Given that corporate health care costs are up over 9 percent in 1990 to more than $150 billion, business leaders are alarmed at the potential for these expenses to eat away at profits and threaten the nation's ability to compete internationally.

A poll conducted by Peter Hart Associates and a group called Nurses of America, which represents four major nursing organizations —the American Nurses' Association, the American Organization of Nurse Executives, the American Association of Colleges of Nurses, and the NLN—demonstrated that the vast majority of Americans believe that bringing costs under control should be a major priority for health care policymakers. By an overwhelming margin (76 percent), Americans were seriously troubled by the rising cost of health care.

According to the poll, Americans cited physician fees as the number one problem, with lab costs ranking second. A substantial proportion of Americans advocated that the replacement of physicians by certified nurses as providers of basic health care services would be a desirable way to cut costs and maintain quality.

Q *What is the rate of increases in health care expenditures in the United States?*

A Health care inflation has been rising at an annual rate of 10.5 percent, dramatically outpacing the rate of inflation in the United States. Since 1960, health care expenditures have increased over 800 percent, growing annually more than twice as fast as general prices.

Most dramatic among the factors influencing these rising health care expenditures are payments for physician services, which continue to spiral upward at untenable rates. In 1989, Medicare reimbursement to physicians rose 18 percent from the year before.

Q *Can nurses alleviate the problem of high costs in health care?*

A Absolutely. Studies have demonstrated that nurses can reduce health care costs in and out of hospitals. In hospitals, nurses can decrease patients' length of stay by: (1) preventing postoperative complications by spending time educating patients prior to surgery; (2) preventing infections frequently acquired in the hospital setting, such as pneumonia or urinary tract infections; and (3) preventing such conditions as phlebitis and pressure necrosis that are caused by inadequate exercise and mobility. Furthermore, new models for structuring hospital nursing services show promising cost-saving results when nurses are positioned as managers and coordinators of patient care.

For years, nurses have been in the forefront of health promotion and preventive care in the community via the Public Health Service and in the provision of home health care, both of which have been shown to dramatically reduce costs. Nurses are instrumental in preventing hospitalization and costly use of acute-care facilities through patient teaching and counseling about nutrition, exercise, and mental and physical health practices.

In addition, in primary care settings nurse practitioners have been found to be far more cost-effective than physicians, while patient satisfaction is greater. Dr. Claire Fagin's review of literature on primary nursing found 84 percent of nurse practitioners' patients gained satisfactory relief from symptoms, compared with 73 percent of physicians' patients.

Other research has demonstrated that nurse practitioners achieve better control of obesity and hypertension in their patients than physicians do. Similarly, nurse-midwives provide safer care at a fraction of the cost of traditional physician services. (A complete compilation of these studies is available from NLN.)

Q What effort has the federal government undertaken to reduce health care costs?

A Spending on health care and social programs has been the prime target of budget reductions. Beginning in the early 1980s, the Reagan administration established a system of paying hospitals that dramatically changed the way the health industry conducted its business.

Under the new payment system, called "Diagnostic Related Groups" (DRGs), providers are paid a certain amount for the patients they treat, according to the diagnosis. With DRGs, institutions are reimbursed prospectively, meaning they receive a set fee established in advance, for each diagnosis.

Although the new payment system has not reduced the aggregate amounts spent on health care, the new method of payment has encouraged competition and, therefore, the evolution of a new health care marketplace, where all types of arrangements are in competition—health maintenance organizations (HMOs), preferred provider organizations (PPOs), community nursing organizations (CNOs), surgicenters, diagnostic centers, and the like.

| Q | **Did the DRG system of hospital reimbursement affect the quality of patient care?**

| A | Absolutely, say consumers. Many noted authorities believe that quality has been seriously affected, and anecdotal reports abound of hospitalized patients receiving compromised care because of scarce resources. Patients are being discharged sooner, when they are more seriously ill. In addition, they are discharged into a disjointed community health care system. The nursing community is advancing the role of the nurse as case manager to alleviate this problem.

The release of hospital mortality data to the public was at the insistence of powerful consumer groups such as the American Association of Retired Persons (AARP), who wanted to be able to monitor quality on their own. This event triggered the prospect of releasing all types of hospital (and physician) data to the public.

Currently, NLN is supporting a model consumer information disclosure act. (Copies are available from NLN.)

| Q | **What has been the net effect of prospective payment?**

| A | In the final analysis, DRGs accomplished little more than shuffling the deck chairs in health care. While many patients endured a lower quality of care, costs in health care have continued to accelerate faster than they did prior to the implementation of DRGs. The reason for costs rising is not because DRGs

themselves are a bad idea, but because they fail to address the real causes of rising costs in health care—such as expensive high-tech equipment, growth in the proportion of elderly, and the rise in physician incomes.

Q *What is the fastest rising component of health care costs, and what is being done about it?*

A Physician fees are the fastest rising component of health care costs. Because physician costs under Medicare Part B have been rising faster than any other segment of the health care economy, Congress has established a Physician Payment Review Commission to focus on this problem. Recently the commission implemented a set of resource-based relative value scales (RBRVSs), a concept developed by William Hsiao and associates from Harvard University.

RBRVS is a zero-based approach to costing out physician services. It uses an index that assigns weight to each medical service; the weights represent the relative amount to be paid for each service on the basis of what it really costs to provide that service, i.e., the resources used. Resources include all the materials and labor needed by an efficient physician to provide a service or procedure, including the physician's own time and effort.

RBRVS will probably create more parity between the rates paid to heart surgeons, for example, and family physicians, since basic health care services are more in demand. The nursing community is currently requesting that the commission examine nursing salaries—as a preliminary step to acquiring reimbursement under Medicare. Thus, when a nurse's activity is the same as a family physician's, for example, in terms of the resources used, the nurse should get reimbursed for the service.

47

Q *Will RBRVS work to bring down costs?*

A It's too early to say, but it has some advantages that indicate it could see greater success than DRGs. For one thing, RBRVS targets the segment of health care spending that rises faster than any other segment: physician fees, which skyrocketed 18 percent in 1989.

Q *Are nurses affected by RBRVS?*

A Yes. Nursing researchers are working on indexing nursing services as well. The most responsible approach to policy change in health care would identify the most appropriate and economically attractive service, regardless of which provider delivers it. RBRVS should examine nursing practices along with physician services and provide incentives for nurses to function as, for example, providers of primary care or case managers. Study after study demonstrates that nurses provide very high quality services at a fraction of the costs.

Q *Do nurses have other ideas for cutting costs?*

A For decades, nurses have advanced a wide variety of proven effective strategies for cutting costs in many areas. Nursing's agenda focuses on providing preventive care, onging services for the chronically ill and aged, home care services, and community health care and education.

Nursing's emphasis on preventive services and health education has been shown to lower overall health costs by contracting the nation's demand for acute care. The benefits of this approach would be most dramatic in the area of pre- and post-natal care, where inexpensive care provided to pregnant women directly lowers the incidence of premature and low birth weight deliveries and thus prevents infant mortality. Many key studies suggest that deploying nurses to provide perinatal care and education would cut costs dramatically.

Public Access to Health Care

Q *Do all Americans have access to the health care services they need?*

A In spite of per capita health expenditures that outrank any other nation in the world, an estimated 37 million Americans have no access to health services at all. One out of four of these are children. These Americans, and many more with only marginal access to health care services, come in contact with our health care delivery system only in dire emergencies—and taxpayers and insurers indirectly foot the bill.

By the time these working Americans show up in the emergency room, it is too late to provide the preventive care, counseling, and early detection that nurses have the expertise and desire to offer. Whenever we have realized success as a nation in providing access to care, it has been nurses who have alleviated the access problem. The Rural Health Services Act of 1977 was a good example. The act reimbursed nurses for the first time in underserved rural areas, and it succeeded in providing significantly greater access to care.

Payment for nursing services through public financing programs could provide a solution to the access problem. Currently, the Senate Finance Committee is considering such a measure to reimburse community nursing centers.

Q *Wouldn't costs skyrocket if all of the nation's two million nurses suddenly started billing the federal government directly for the services they provide?*

A Yes. We do not advocate reimbursing all nurses—but a critical mass of case managers, clinical specialists, and nurse practitioners should be included.

Q *What is managed care?*

A Managed care is a mechanism whereby purchasers of care—employers and the federal government—design the best package of services at the lowest cost. Managed care arrangements emphasize the appropriateness of care and reduced hospital stays, as well as cost reduction.

Q *If direct reimbursement for some nursing services makes so much sense in terms of cost and quality, why don't we have it?*

A Politics. Barriers resulting from battles over "turf" continue to beset the nursing profession. Some of the most formidable opposition comes from organized medicine. Many physicians are threatened by the notion of nurses as primary care providers because they perceive this as competition and a threat to their practice.

The growing surplus of physicians no doubt intensifies this situation, as physicians strive to hold their share of the market. Despite some successful collaborating arrangements between individual nurses and physicians, barriers to third-party reimbursement for nurses are intensified at state and national levels. The American Medical Association's (AMA's) political action committees and well-established networks on both national and state levels often present obstacles to nurses working to overcome barriers to reimbursement in the legislative arena.

50

Q *Aren't many nurses currently reimbursed for their services?*

A Yes. Nurses have achieved a great deal of success through enactment of state legislation that allows for direct third-party reimbursement for nursing. As of January 1986, approximately 26 states had passed legislation providing insurance for nursing services. Many other states have pending legislation. Nurse-midwives, nurse anesthetists, and many psychiatric nurses are currently reimbursed for their services. (For an up-to-date list of the status of state legislation on nursing practice, contact NLN.)

Q *Why is third-party reimbursement for nursing practice important for consumers?*

A Consumers have the right to choose the health care providers and practitioners they prefer. If the chosen practitioner is qualified to deliver health care but is ineligible for third-party reimbursement because of public or private reimbursement policies, then consumers are in effect prohibited from deciding who will provide their health care. Thus the movement to obtain third-party reimbursement for nurses is of importance not only to nurses themselves but also to consumers, who are entitled to access to and benefits of nursing care. Without policies that allow for reimbursement for nursing care, there is a disincentive for consumers to seek care from nurses in expanded or entrepreneurial roles. Further, surveys of the American public have demonstrated that consumers would support an expansion of nursing services if they knew it would lower their health care costs.

The Tri-Council, composed of the NLN, the ANA, the American Organization of Nurse Executives, and the American Association of Colleges of Nursing, conducted its own survey of attitudes of the American public. The survey demonstrated clearly that the public believes nurses are underutilized and should be given more responsibility and authority.

51

Q *What types of nursing services do insurance companies pay for?*

A Some insurance carriers have covered nursing services for quite some time. Company policy is affected by the laws or regulations pertaining to third-party reimbursement for nurses in that particular state. A number of insurance policies allow for reimbursement of nurse-midwives, nurse practitioners, and psychiatric care delivered by a nurse. Nurses should urge patients to inquire about the provisions of their policies.

Currently, many policies allow for reimbursement to nurses as long as the services being paid for are normally covered and allowed under the state's nurse practice act. For example, if psychotherapy is covered by the insurance policy, and the state law allows for nurses to provide psychotherapy services, then psychotherapy provided by a nurse is an allowable expense under that policy. On the other hand, if visits for health promotion and disease prevention are not covered by an insurance company, then no matter how broad the state's reimbursement laws are, nurses cannot be reimbursed for those services.

Q *Are any nurses currently reimbursed under Medicare?*

A Yes. Nurse-midwives are eligible for reimbursement under Medicare, but few Medicare patients require nurse-midwifery services. Under the Rural Health Clinics Act of 1977, nurse practitioners providing care to Medicare patients in designated rural clinics are eligible for reimbursement. In addition, the Omnibus Reconciliation Act of 1987 created demonstration projects to provide payment on a prepaid, capitated basis for community nursing and ambulatory care furnished to Medicare beneficiaries. These are the only instances where nurses can be reimbursed under Medicare.

| Q | What kind of nurses would consumers make appointments to see if we had a system of direct reimbursement? |

| A | Primarily nurse practitioners, clinical specialists, and case managers. Examples include nurses in community health centers and home care and at hospitals providing special services such as case management. For example, nurse-midwives, nurse anesthetists, clinical specialists, and nurses in advanced practice would provide physical assessments, health information counseling to prevent disease, and nursing management of chronic disease states. |

| Q | What if my child had a cold, or I needed an annual physical? |

| A | You could take your child to a pediatric nurse practitioner. Nurse practitioners (NPs) are nurses who provide basic primary care, including history taking, physical assessment, patient education, screening and management of routine health problems, prescribing medications within the scope of their practice, counseling, and referral to other health care providers as needed. |

Nurse practitioners obtain preparation beyond their basic education, usually as part of a master's program in nursing, and specialize in one area, such as pediatrics, geriatrics, psychiatric-mental health, family practice, or midwifery.

The quality of care delivered by nurse practitioners rivals that of physicians, and in several respects exceeds it. According to a 1986 study by the Office of Technology Assessment, nurse practitioners providing primary care services achieved substantially higher marks from consumers than physician counterparts on patient communication and follow up, and cost less.

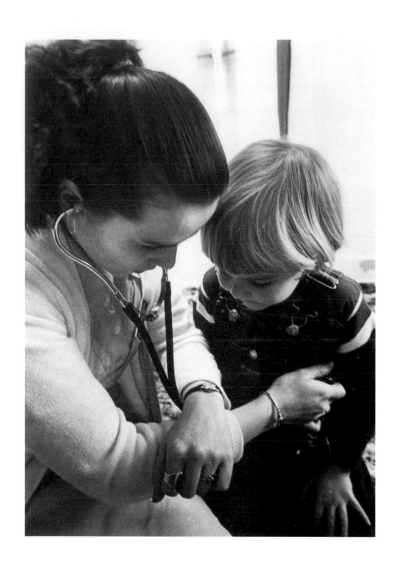

Q *How is a nurse practitioner different from a registered nurse?*

A The NP movement started in the early 1960s under the leadership of Loretta Ford, PhD, RN, and Henry Silver, MD. Each state regulates NPs through the state's nurse practice act. In some states, NPs were able to practice without significant changes in existing statutes. In states that prohibit nurses from engaging in diagnosis and prescribing treatment, NPs cannot practice without new statutory authority. The response in these states has been either to replace previous statutes with new definitions of nursing roles or to amend existing law to accommodate expanded nursing practice.

Reimbursement also remains a major obstacle to the use of NPs. However, federal legislation in 1977 paved the way for future revisions in third-party reimbursement for NPs: the Rural Health Clinics Act enabled NPs to be reimbursed under Medicare and Medicaid for the services they provided in certified rural health clinics. The bill provided for direct third-party reimbursement for NP services in underserved areas, without requiring an accompanying physician's signature, as long as the NP services were authorized under state legislation.

There is still considerable variation in the type of reimbursement that third-party payers offer for NP services. Some states and third-party payers allow for third-party reimbursement of NPs as one of many types of nursing services. Others have policies that focus solely on NPs.

Q Can nurses manage normal pregnancy and delivery without direct physician input?

A Nurse-midwives can. A nurse-midwife is a registered nurse who is a specialist in maternal and child health. Nurse-midwives care for women throughout the course of normal pregnancies, deliver babies, and deliver primary health care to women and normal newborns. A nurse-midwife who completes a course of graduate study and passes a national certifying exam becomes a certified nurse-midwife (CNM).

Approximately 3,000 CNMs care for women across the nation in clinical collaboration with physicians. CNMs may be employed by hospitals or work in group or independent practice. Nurse-midwifery practice has become increasingly accepted by consumers as a cost-effective alternative to traditional medical practice.

Like nurse practitioners, nurse-midwives have been shown to provide a very high quality of care, often exceeding that of obstetricians.

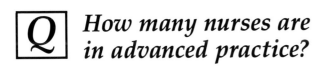 **Do any nurses currently have hospital admitting privileges?**

A Yes. Certain advanced level nurses practice in hospitals, and consumers can choose among them the way they choose among physicians. Two of the most common advanced level nurses in hospitals are nurse anesthetists and nurse-midwives. Extensive research exists attesting to the high quality and cost-effectiveness of their services.

In 1983, the District of Columbia was the first U.S. jurisdiction to pass legislation granting nurses clinical admitting privileges and staff membership. Since then, other states have introduced legislation expanding nursing's scope of practice. Despite advances such as these in the legislative arena, nurses still face obstacles to independent practice through the regulatory process and other activities initiated by organized medicine.

Q **How many nurses are in advanced practice?**

A It is estimated that 0.2 percent of the nurses in the United States are nurse-midwives, 1.8 percent are clinical specialists, 1.1 percent are nurse clinicians, 1.3 percent are nurse practitioners, and 1.0 percent are certified nurse anesthetists. These numbers are growing as state reimbursement laws eliminate payment barriers and more nurses are willing to make use of the opportunities afforded by the increasingly competitive health care system to risk an entrepreneurial venture. Growing consumer awareness of and appreciation for nurse practitioners, midwives, and psychotherapists also contribute to the proliferation of nurses in expanded practice.

Q *Can nurses ever practice independently of physicians in spite of the limitations on direct reimbursement?*

A Absolutely. By virtue of their education and knowledge base, nurses are qualified to practice in a wide range of settings, such as clinics, day-care centers, schools, housing projects for the elderly, and private nursing practice. In these settings, nurses perform a wide range of functions, including screening for diseases, patient education, psychosocial counseling, and promoting self-care.

However, despite documented consumer satisfaction with and increasing demand for independent nursing care, formidable barriers to practice have limited the number of nurses able to practice independently. Principal among these are restrictive state practice acts and insufficient third-party coverage for autonomous nursing care. In many states, nurses have fought successfully to eliminate the restrictions on their practice, thereby giving consumers greater access to nursing care.

Q *In what ways is nursing care preferable to medical care?*

A In ambulatory settings, patients need nursing care more often than medical care in order to maintain the best possible health status. For example, patients with chronic illnesses such as diabetes or heart disease often need education and guidance to help them comply with medication, treatment regimens, and life-style adjustments. They also need counseling abut the chronicity and psychosocial aspects of their conditions.

Similarly, infants and children are generally well and not in need of acute medical care.

To grow and develop to the best of their potential, they require periodic developmental and physical assessments and screening for abnormal conditions. Often their parents require counseling and guidance about the stages of child development and parenting concerns such as toilet training, sibling rivalry, disciplining, or school problems. These are services that can be rendered by nurses with advanced preparation as pediatric nurse practitioners. These families would then need medical care from a pediatrician only for management of acute episodic illnesses, such as pneumonia or other complex medical situations or emergencies.

The major tools of medical practice are drugs and surgery—needed to treat disease. The tools of medical science do not emphasize the holistic aspects of health care. Nursing's interest, however, lies in the complete person: individuals at home, in the family, at work, or in the community.

Nursing care is preferable to medical care when patients are most concerned with health promotion, education in areas such as medication and nutrition, and learning about self-help and other ways that they can actively assume responsibility for their own health. There is a great deal of overlap between medical and nursing practice, and nurses and physicians often collaborate to offer patients a full range of services.

In short, whenever the health care needs of a particular population focus on disease prevention, patient education, and health maintenance, nursing care is appropriate. When a patient is acutely ill and needs disease–focused care, or presents with a complicated condition, then the services of a physician are in order.

Q *If I choose to see a nurse for primary care, how can I be sure that I'm receiving high quality, cost-effective care?*

A As with any provider, the patient has the right to a complete understanding of all procedures, decisions, and options available and to have questions answered and fears alleviated. Therefore, one indicator of quality would be customer satisfaction with the information and treatment provided and the outcome of the services provided.

The nursing community is currently working toward the standardization of criteria to identify excellence in practice through the newly created Board of Nursing Specialties. In the near future, the public will be able to look for certification as a measure of the clinician's quality. At present, certification standards are too varied and lack sufficient consistency to have meaning to the public.

Quality in Health Care

Q *How do you measure quality?*

A Until fairly recently, policymakers measured quality in much the same way judges measure obscenity: they knew it when they saw it. In the case of health care quality, more often than not they knew when they didn't see it. Claims of malpractice offered episodic and frequently contradictory rules on what does and does not constitute bad quality practice.

Presently, however, the need to cut costs in a beleaguered delivery system and chilling incidences of poor quality have led to increasing efforts on the part of policymakers to define quality.

Initial attempts at identifying measures of quality focused on hospital mortality rates and rates of cure. But such factors, though important, measure only a small fraction of the health care services delivered every day in the nation. Efforts to measure more sophisticated aspects of quality, such as judging the caliber of physician services or the quality of surgical procedures, or even nursing care of the chronically ill are currently ongoing.

$\boxed{Q}$ *If maximizing well being, not just curing, is a goal of care—for instance, home care services for a chronically ill individual or a checkup for a healthy person—is it possible to measure and ensure the quality of care delivered?*

$\boxed{A}$ Absolutely. New models for measuring patient outcomes emerge every day, especially in nursing research. The most promising innovation in defining and ensuring high quality care is a national project generously funded by the W. K. Kellogg Foundation and conducted by the Community Health Accreditation Program (CHAP) of the NLN. The aim of the project is to identify consumer-oriented outcomes of care. For the first time ever, *consumer's* definitions of quality will be included in the quality outcome measures in the home care industry, and eventually the accreditation process will be too.

CHAP, with a unique governing board consisting of nurses, physicians, insurers, and consumers, sets high quality standards for home care that reflect the needs of all participants in the delivery of services, from the patient to the provider to the payer. It may seem like common sense that patients have a valuable perspective on what constitutes good care, but CHAP is the first accrediting body to consider the consumer viewpoint.

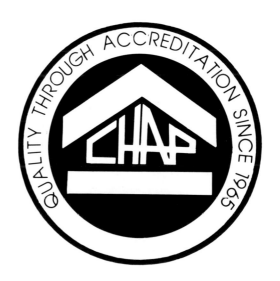

Q *How does a discerning consumer choose the highest quality provider?*

A Despite the importance of choosing a physician, hospital, nursing home, home care agency, or other service, little information is available to help the public discern between competing providers. What quality data that does exist is almost always unavailable to the public.

CHAP is the only accrediting body in the nation with a policy of full public disclosure of vital quality information. CHAP offers consumers full data on the quality of care delivered at accredited agencies.

Q *Has the federal government done anything to promote public disclosure of quality information?*

A Yes, and consumers have advanced this agenda. The Health Care Financing Administration (HCFA) has identified several quality indicators, particularly mortality data. In an unprecedented step that angered many in the delivery system, notably physician and hospital groups, the first of these data were released in December 1987 on 735,000 deaths among Medicare patients treated at nearly 6,000 acute-care hospitals during 1986. Of the 5,971 hospitals listed, 5,825 had death rates that were either within the predicted range or below it. The 146 hospitals remaining had mortality rates above expectations.

The release of this data flew in the face of business as usual in health care which closely guards the confidentiality of quality data. Nonetheless, as powerful as the health care industry is, it cannot compete with the collective power of American consumers, who have grown increasingly vigilant in demanding higher quality care and the information to identify it.

Consumer groups believe the data will help to improve the quality of health care. Though the mortality rates should not be used as an absolute measure of quality, the information can screen for potential problems within institutions and consumers lobbied successfully for access to it. Though HCFA is criticized because its mortality rates do not take into consideration the patient's severity index, we can expect to see more of these data as a trend in measuring quality.

Furthermore, HCFA will use its data on 10 million hospital records and 250 million physician services provided each year to measure medical effectiveness. Though decisions on patient treatment will remain with physicians and nurses, HCFA plans to eventually rank treatments by effectiveness on different kinds of patients.

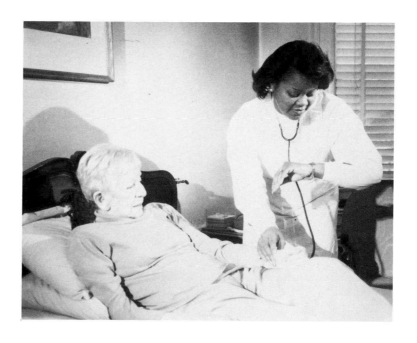

Q *Why did HCFA choose mortality data as a measure of quality?*

A Essentially, it was the easiest to obtain and measure. HCFA, under pressure to measure the quality of services provided to patients receiving Medicare, decided to use mortality rates as empirical data. Mortality data were accessible through the files collected at HCFA and were measured against a range of predicted mortality, factoring in age, sex, diagnosis, comorbidity, chronic conditions, prior hospitalizations, and hospital transfer.

Most experts concede that mortality rates should not be used as an absolute measure of quality. The information is not intended to be used as a direct measure of quality of care but could be used as a screening tool to identify hospitals' strengths and weaknesses. One shortcoming of the study is that it did not take severity of illness into account.

Q *What quality indicators will HCFA use for future measurement in the health care industry?*

A HCFA has been in the process of collecting data on the effectiveness of certain treatments on patient outcomes. The objective of these studies is to assess the impact of these interventions: (1) on mortality and morbidity; (2) on the use of inpatient and ambulatory services as measures of morbidity; (3) on the use of supportive services as measures of disability; and (4) on overall expenditures for medical care alternatives after adjustment for the condition of the patient, including severity of illness.

Ultimately, this information will be useful in guiding the choices of specific treatments.

Q *What is the state of research on patient outcome measures as a means of improving quality health care?*

A The newest agency within the U.S. Public Health Service, the Agency for Health Care Policy and Research, has created initiatives to encourage the development of new methods for assessing the effectiveness of medical interventions and the outcomes of medical care. It is hoped that these new methods and the resulting assessments will lead to the development of clinical practice guidelines. Ultimately, improved information will result, for both patients and providers, in better and more effective clinical decision making and possibly reduced health care expenditures, thereby improving the quality of health care services.

Q *What about the quality of care in nursing homes? Does HCFA have a plan to release quality indicators for the nursing home industry?*

A Yes, HCFA has released to the public information about the performance of over 15,000 nursing homes in the country participating in Medicare and Medicaid. The initiative contained information on each facility's resident population and performance obtained from on-site inspections conducted by state survey agencies.

This information will serve as a tool to improve consumer ability to make informed decisions in selecting nursing homes.

The Nursing Shortage

Q *Is there still a nursing shortage?*

A Yes. The current shortage of nurses cuts across all health care settings and all nursing practice settings. Even though NLN data (*New York Times*, December 28, 1990) demonstrate an increase in 1990 enrollments to schools of nursing of 14 percent, the nationwide nursing shortage persists and will grow exponentially in the future if measures are not adopted to alleviate it. The Secretary's Commission on the nursing shortage found that the shortage cuts across all health care settings and all regions of the nation, although it is most acute in rural and inner city areas and in the long-term care industry.

The commission discovered that the key to solving the shortage lies not in increasing the numbers of nurses alone, but in more appropriate utilization of RNs. If nurses are used more effectively, not only will institutions gain hours of valuable nursing expertise, but more appropriate utilization will also enhance the attractiveness of nursing as an exciting career option to new entrants into the field.

Another key commission finding cited the need for enhanced long-term career opportunities. Nurses need a path for career development that includes growing opportunity for higher levels of authority, autonomy, and salary.

As the commission articulated in its report, and as hundreds of other panels and studies concur, the shortage results from the escalating demand for highly skilled nursing services. As the population ages and high-technology innovations enable increasing numbers of chronically ill people to survive on life-support systems or in other

67

long-term states of dependency, the need for skilled nursing care grows precariously. According to the commission, RN vacancy rates have hit an all-time high of 18.9 percent in nursing homes, 12.9 percent in home health agencies, 12 percent in hospitals, and 10.5 percent in HMOs.

| Q | *What is causing an increased demand for registered nurses?*

| A | Misutilization of registered nurses has created the tremendous demand. In a workload management study undertaken by the Army and Navy, only 26 percent of a registered nurse's eight-hour work shift was devoted to direct patient care. The remainder of time was spent completing clerical work and transporting patients and laboratory specimens. Furthermore, most institutions find nurses the most versatile and cost-effective providers of health care services to employ.

Nurses have a broad knowledge base and are able to function efficiently in a variety of capacities (i.e., as nurse's aides on the low skill end of the scale, and at the high end of the scale, nurses can perform many of the tasks that physicians perform). Because of this versatility, health care employers hire registered nurses over other health care providers, and usually at a lower cost, creating an increase in demand.

Another factor creating greater demand has been increased patient acuity levels in hospitals as a result of cost containment strategies. In response to shifting demands resulting from the introduction of DRGs, from 1984 to 1986 alone, there was an increase in nurse-patient ratios from 8.6 RNs to 9.6 RNs per 100 patients. Today, nurse-patient ratios remain high, 9.9 RNs per 100 patients.

In addition, sicker patients are being discharged from the hospital, requiring more nurses to meet these patients' home health care needs. An expansion in technology and services in the health care marketplace has also created more opportunities and jobs for nurses.

Q Are enough nurses being prepared to meet the demands of the health care system in the future?

A Serious declines in enrollments in schools of nursing from 1983 to 1988 will compound the nursing supply crisis for future years. NLN data has begun to show a change in direction for nursing school enrollments. In 1989, enrollments to all basic RN schools of nursing increased 8.9 percent. Preliminary NLN data for 1990 show an increase of 14 percent in enrollments. In addition, 1989 data show that associate degree enrollments increased 10.6 percent, diploma enrollments increased 8.3 percent, and baccalaureate degree enrollments increased 6.8 percent. This represents a total of approximately 202,000 students. Despite the current enrollment increases, the downward trend in enrollments from 1983 through 1988 will have a lasting impact.

The Department of Health and Human Services *Seventh Report to the President and Congress on the Status of Health Personnel in the United States* projected requirements for full-time equivalent registered nurses with baccalaureate, master's, and doctoral degrees are about twice the projected supply for the years 2000 and 2010. For nurses with associate degrees, the supply is about two times higher than the projected requirements in 2000 and then begins to level off in 2010 and 2020.

One estimate cited in the Institute of Medicine study projected that the demand for nurses with master's degrees would reach

256,000 by the early 1990s, while the actual supply is projected at less than half that number—only 112,400. The supply of doctorally prepared nurses was predicted to reach only 5,600 by the early 1990s, in contrast to a projected demand for nearly 14,000.

| Q | *Where are most nurses employed?* |

| A | Of those employed in nursing, an estimated 68 percent work in hospitals. The second largest group of employers is ambulatory care settings, where 7.7 percent of nurses are employed. Proportions of nurses in other employment settings are as follows: 6.8 percent in community and public health, 6.6 percent in nursing home and extended care facilities, 1.8 percent in nursing education, 2.9 percent in schools, 1.2 percent in private duty nursing, 0.8 percent self-employed, and 1.3 percent in occupational health (Figure 1).

| Q | *What is the average salary of registered nurses?* |

| A | As of 1988, the median annual salary of all registered nurses employed full time was $28,383. The average salary of staff nurses was $26,263. Those in administrative positions earned $34,564, a difference of $8,300, or 32 percent more than the average for a staff nurse.

Nurses employed in staff nurse positions in occupational health settings and in hospitals have the highest average annual salaries for staff level positions, $27,389 and $27,196, respectively. Staff nurses in ambulatory care settings have the lowest salaries, $21,528, followed by staff nurses in nursing homes and other extended care facilities, $22,381.

Figure 1. Field of Employment of Registered Nurses, March 1988

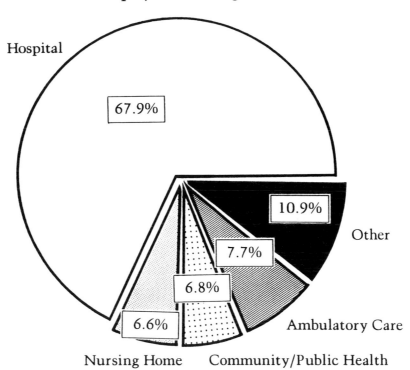

Source: DN, National Sample Survey.

The average salary for staff nurses in nursing homes showed the largest increase between November 1984 and March 1988, 23 percent. The average salary for hospital staff nurses increased 21 percent. School health nurses' and public health/community health nurses' average salaries showed the smallest increases.

Nurses working in community health and long-term care settings do not always receive salaries that are competitive with those of their colleagues in hospitals. However, this is changing as non-acute-care agencies seek to attract qualified nurses who are increasingly in demand as care becomes more complex.

For nursing faculty, the average annual salary is related to highest earned credential, years of experience, and whether the faculty member's appointment is for a calendar or academic year. For 1988, the mean salary for a full professor with a doctoral degree in a baccalaureate or higher-degree program was $54,500.

Q *If nurses' salaries are comparable to those of other professions, why does the nursing profession state that nurses are underpaid?*

A It is true that starting salaries for nurses are comparable to other professionals. It is also true that some nurses in top level positions make substantial salaries. But on the average, after five to seven years on the job, a nurse's salary peaks at just over $29,000, or a 39 percent increase for a lifetime of work. This is very low as compared to accountants who receive a 200 percent increase over a lifetime of work. This salary compression deters nurses from lifelong careers in nursing.

Q *What factors related to their work setting are most important to nurses?*

A Adequate staffing, with ancillary staff to assist with non-nursing functions, is cited as important to nurses. Nurses are very concerned with the need for low patient-to-RN ratios and stress the importance of taking into account the type and complexity of patients' needs for care. Other factors reported as important are career growth, salaries, benefits, flexible work hours, educational access, and mobility.

Q *What are key functions of the registered nurse in the hospital?*

A It is the responsibility of the nursing staff to provide 24-hour care for hospitalized patients. This means that the registered nurse works with patients and their families to make sure that patients receive the appropriate treatments and medications, are relieved of pain and discomfort, are encouraged to engage in self-care activities as much as possible, and are kept informed of their rights and responsibilities as consumers of health care.

Most important, it is the nurse who is responsible for the full range of patient care needs, including the physiological and psychosocial responses to illness. This includes counseling and guiding patients and their families as they adjust to the illness and learn how to cope with the stress and disruption of hospitalization.

The nurse is the primary patient educator, explaining the reason for treatments and leading patients toward an optimal state of health and well-being by giving them as much information as possible about their condition.

Nurses also serve as coordinators for the many different facets of hospital care and for discharge planning, ensuring that the patient can continue to receive necessary care at home or in another setting.

Q How can patients tell how much they are paying for nursing care?

A Historically, hospitals have included nursing costs as part of the room-and-board charge instead of identifying them separately. This is changing rapidly, however, as significant numbers of hospitals have begun to cost out nursing care for internal purposes or to include a separate nursing charge in their patients' bills.

Several recent studies have indicated that nursing costs account for approximately 20 percent of the average bill. It is important for hospitals to have precise information about the costs and utilization of nursing personnel in order to make the most appropriate and cost-effective decisions about assignment of nurses and to determine to what extent nursing care units are revenue or cost centers for the institution.

73

Figure 2. The Increasing Size of the Elderly Population Age 65 and Older, in Millions and Percent of Population

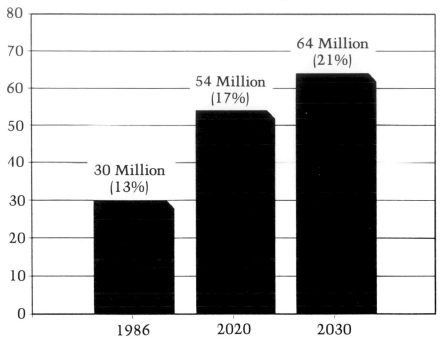

Through careful research, nurses across the country have made progress in identifying the costs of nursing care for inpatients. Some studies link the cost of nursing care with nursing diagnosis, others with nursing patient classification systems, utilization of nursing services, severity of illness, or length of stay.

In the future, as the methodology for costing out nursing service improves, more patients will receive specific information on their hospital bills regarding the costs of the nursing care they received.

$\boxed{Q}$ *In what settings will there be the greatest future demand for nurses?*

$\boxed{A}$ In anticipation of a more severely ill case mix in acute-care settings, as well as accelerated use of HMOs, community nursing organizations, home health, and other types of community-based care, there is a general consensus among manpower experts that nurses will be in particularly high demand through the year 2000. With pressure from the federal government to cut health care costs, home care as a cost-effective alternative will most likely become the mainstay in health care. Home care is currently the fastest growing segment of health care.

The "graying" of America will require greater demands on nursing. It is projected that the over-65 population will constitute 17 percent in the year 2020, as opposed to 13 percent of the population in 1986 (Figure 2).

The recently passed legislation on Nursing Home Reform, which amended Title XVIII of the Social Security Act, has increased requirements in skilled nursing facilities to employ a registered nurse at least eight hours a day, seven days a week. This requirement will increase demands for long-term care registered nurses. Shifting patterns of care resulting from the Medicare prospective payment system (PPS) have reduced total inpatient hospital days since the inception of the PPS in 1983. This has caused the "sicker and quicker" phenomenon requiring increased demands for registered nurses in community health and home care.

| Q | *What types of education will be needed for future nurses?* |

| A | Graduate-prepared clinical nurse specialists and nurse practitioners will be needed to deliver primary care to high-risk populations (the elderly, the very young, and those from low socioeconomic groups) and to improve access to care in underserved regions. Numerous studies document the cost savings, patient satisfaction, and improvements in health status that can result from primary care rendered by nurse practitioners.

Graduate-prepared nurse administrators will continue to be in great demand to meet the challenges of the health care system. These nurses need sound knowledge of computers, financing, budgeting, and management in order to administer nursing services in the new financially driven, fiscally restrained environment.

Nurses with graduate degrees are also needed in nursing education. Among nursing faculty, 66.6 percent have a master's degree as their highest degree earned; only 32 percent are doctorally prepared. Federal support is needed to promote education of nurse faculty, of whom a smaller proportion are graduate-prepared than in most other professions. NLN data show that in 1988 over 750 full-time nursing faculty positions remained unfilled nationwide, with over 500 of those positions in baccalaureate and higher-degree nursing programs.

Q How does the surplus of physicians affect the demand for nurses?

A As nurses strive to become independent providers of primary care, their attempts to deliver more affordable, high-quality care are being increasingly challenged by physicians seeking work in the same settings. As consumer acceptance of nurses as primary care providers increases, the demand for nurses will increase, and the competition between nurses and physicians is likely to accelerate as well.

The potential for competition between nurses and physicians is demonstrated by a 1984 AMA resolution that opposed legislation expanding nonphysicians' practice. This resolution typifies the attitude AMA has held on the expansion of nursing practice. The 1984 resolution assisted state medical associations to systematically block legislation authorizing independent practice, prescribing privileges, mandated third-party reimbursement, and other expanded practices of providers such as nurse practitioners, nurse-midwives, and nurse anesthetists.

A proposal passed by the 1988 AMA House of Delegates was for a new level of caregiver, the registered care technologist (RCT). This proposal is further evidence that organized medicine wants control over all aspects of the health care delivery system with all providers held accountable to medicine. This competitive edge could further complicate nursing's ability to provide comprehensive health care services to people in need of nursing services, not to mention the unnecessary proliferation of categories of direct caregivers.

The latest report from the AMA Board of Trustees came in early 1990 regarding independent nursing practice models. AMA concludes it will continue to monitor federal and state independent nursing practice models and encourage statutory changes so that physicians may retain their intermediary responsibilities for direct patient care.

The physician surplus, combined with organized medicine's attempt to block legislation authorizing expansion of nursing practice, has created conflict between nurses and physicians in the legislative arena. Fortunately, with consumer support as a contributing factor, nurses have succeeded in legitimizing their expanded roles through legislation. Examples are legislation passed in the District of Columbia granting clinical privileges to certain kinds of nurses, as well as the growing number of states with new legislation mandating direct third-party reimbursement for nursing care.

Q *Have increasing opportunities for women to enter other professions affected the supply of nurses?*

A One of nursing's greatest challenges in the future will be to recruit bright, talented women and men into the profession. Recruitment into nursing has become increasingly difficult as women are lured into professions perceived to be more prestigious and lucrative. In 1972, women constituted 39 percent of all professional workers; by 1990, that share had risen to 45 percent. From 1980 to 1990, the number of self–employed women (the majority of whom are sole proprietors) increased 30 percent.

A dramatic growth in size of the female segment of the labor force has occurred among women age 25 to 54. By 1990, their labor force participation rate had reached nearly 73 percent, an increase of more than 18 percentage points over the previous decade. This expanded pool increases the opportunities for nursing schools to recruit potential students. However, with many other careers open to women that were not readily available to them 20 or 30 years ago, competition for these potential students stiffens.

Q *What other factors will affect the supply of nurses in the future?*

A The traditional college-age population from which nursing historically drew most of its applicants peaked in size in 1980 at close to 9 million. There is a 26 percent decrease in the number of 18-year-olds today in the United States, a trend that is expected to persist until the mid-1990s. Recent data show that adult learners, students over age 25 who attend college at least part-time, are the most rapidly growing group of college students. This means that nursing, as well as other professions, will be able to draw from this older student population.

In addition, in recent years the amount of student aid available from the federal government has declined dramatically. For example, the cost of a college education increased 69 percent from 1985 to 1990, while federal assistance for higher education dropped by nearly 60 percent in the same time period.

The Nursing Student Loan Program administered by the Bureau of Health Professions has not received any new federal appropriations since 1983. Since then, it has functioned as an approximately $18 million revolving fund, in which loan repayments subsidize the new loans granted. This freeze on new funds, coupled with cutbacks in other areas of public funding for nursing education, has meant that considerably less funding is available to nursing students, making nursing student recruitment more difficult.

| Q | **What is the unemployment rate for nurses compared with the economywide unemployment rate?**

| A | The unemployment rate among RNs has declined in recent years to a record low of 0.9 percent, considerably lower than the national average, which in the best of times is five times that size (Figure 3). It is interesting that a 1984 federal government survey of nurses indicated that nurses are remaining in the work force longer than they did in the past. This may be because of the changing nature of employment for women in general: more women enter the work force and stay employed through their childbearing years, and more women return to work after raising children.

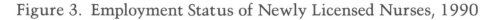

Figure 3. Employment Status of Newly Licensed Nurses, 1990

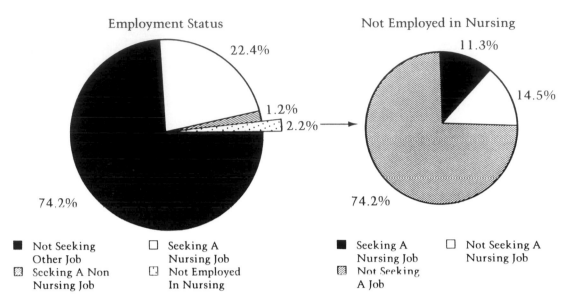

	Employment Status		Not Employed in Nursing
Not Seeking Other Job	Seeking A Nursing Job	Seeking A Nursing Job	Not Seeking A Nursing Job
Seeking A Non Nursing Job	Not Employed In Nursing	Not Seeking A Job	

Q What is the Institute of Medicine study on nursing?

A It was a two-year congressionally mandated study, completed in 1983 by the Institute of Medicine of the National Academy of Sciences. The full name of the study is *Nursing and Nursing Education: Public Policies and Private Actions.* The study was prompted by the controversy over whether further federal outlays for nursing education and research would be needed to ensure an adequate supply of nurses. The study's 21 recommendations have served as the basis for subsequent policy recommendations regarding the nursing profession. Most notably, recommendation No. 8 says that the federal government should expand its support of graduate nursing education to increase the number of nurses with master's and doctoral degrees in nursing. Recommendation No. 18 states that the federal government should establish an organizational entity to place nursing research in the mainstream of scientific investigation. This recommendation gave impetus to the arguments in favor of establishment of the National Center for Nursing Research at the National Institutes of Health.

| Q | What is the National Commission on Nursing?

| A | In December of 1987, in response to reports of widespread difficulties recruiting and retaining registered nurses, Secretary of Health and Human Services, Otis R. Bowen, established the Secretary's Commission on Nursing. This 25-member public advisory panel was given the charge to advise the Secretary on problems related to the recruitment and retention of RNs, and to develop recommendations on how the public and private sectors can work together to address these problems and implement immediate and long-range solutions for enhancing the adequacy of the supply of RNs.

| Q | What is the Commission on the National Nursing Shortage?

| A | In February of 1990, the Secretary of Health and Human Services, Dr. Louis Sullivan, appointed a commission to assist in implementing the recommendations of the 1988 Secretary's Commission on Nursing. Chaired by Gloria Smith, PhD, RN, the Commission on the National Nursing Shortage will advise the Secretary on specific projects to optimally use available resources and expertise. Recommended projects will target recruitment and educational pathways, retention and career development, restructuring nursing services and effective utilization of nursing personnel, data collection and analysis requirements, and information systems and related technology in nursing.

The charge given to this 25-member, public advisory panel was to advise the Secretary on problems related to the recruitment and retention of RNs and develop recommendations on how the public and private sectors can work together to address these problems and implement immediate and long-range solutions for enhancing the adequacy of the supply of RNs.

Nursing Education

What educational preparation is required to practice nursing?

A Graduates of baccalaureate nursing education programs in colleges and universities; hospital-based diploma programs; and associate degree programs, most of which are housed in community and junior colleges, are currently eligible to take the RN licensure examination. Graduates of practical/vocational nursing education programs in vocational and technical schools are eligible to take the LPN/LVN licensure examination.

During the past two decades, there has been a decided shift toward educational preparation for nursing in institutions of higher learning. The number of baccalaureate and associate degree programs, and the proportion of nursing students enrolled in these programs, have increased dramatically, while enrollments have declined in diploma programs, long the predominant form of educational preparation for nursing.

During the late 1960s and the 1970s, federal policy was aimed at boosting overall nursing manpower and eradicating a chronic shortage of nurses through support for all types of undergraduate nursing education. In recent years, government studies have pointed repeatedly to a growing shortage of nurses with baccalaureate and graduate degrees. Federal funding is now broad-based for all advanced and specialized areas of preparation and all levels of education. Also, new monies are available for national nurse recruitment centers, faculty development, and educational mobility and access for nurses wishing to advance their education.

| **Q** | *What is the future direction of nursing education?* |

| **A** | Unfortunately, there is no consensus among nursing organizations in support of a particular path of education for professional nursing practice. Therefore, it is incumbent upon the nursing community to examine the nation's future needs for all types of nursing care and project how many and what kinds of nurses will be needed. In this way, educational institutions and government bodies could make plans based on projected demand for nursing care.

NLN is currently conducting a study to differentiate the competencies of graduates and the outcomes achieved from various types of programs. The results of this undertaking should be helpful in guiding the education and utilization of all nurses.

| **Q** | *How many nursing education programs of each type are there in the United States?* |

| **A** | As of 1989, there were 630 baccalaureate programs. Of these, 488 were so-called generic programs, or programs mainly for students without prior nursing education. The remaining 142 programs were RN-completion programs for registered nurses with associate degrees or diplomas who wish to complete their baccalaureate degrees. Also in 1989, there were 812 associate degree programs and 157 diploma schools.

According to 1989 NLN data, 212 institutions offer master's programs in nursing. An additional 47 offer doctoral programs.

Q *What are current enrollments in nursing schools? What have been the enrollment trends over the past ten years?*

A Enrollments in baccalaureate programs dropped from 129,111 in 1980 to 116,539 in 1989, a 9.7 percent decline. The most significant increase within this population was for RNs with diplomas or associate degrees returning for baccalaureate degrees. This number grew from 33,253 in 1980 to 41,674 in 1989, a growth of 25.3 percent.

Associate degree enrollments increased 12.9 percent from 94,060 in 1980 to 106,175 in 1989.

Diploma enrollments showed a 50.2 percent decline over that same ten-year period, from 41,048 to 20,418.

Enrollments of nurses in graduate programs continue to increase in response to the continued demand for master's and doctorally prepared nurses. Between 1980 and 1989, enrollments in master's programs grew 50 percent, from 15,053 to 22,587. Doctoral enrollments, more than doubled for the 1980 to 1989 period, from 1,019 to 2,417.

On December 28, 1990, the *New York Times* reported on the basis of data from NLN's Division of Research, "big gain in nursing students lifts hopes amid a shortage."

Q *How do most nursing students finance their education?*

A Most nursing students rely on a variety of resources and go into considerable debt to finance their education. In the 1970s, federal assistance was a major source of support. Now, although federal funding has diminished and is predicted to drop even more in the future because of the federal budget deficit, the federal government still provides assistance in the form of loans or traineeships for nursing students. Student loans are available for undergraduate and graduate nursing students; traineeships are targeted for graduate nursing students. Both are given to nursing schools, which then grant the funding to eligible students. Federal loans for all nursing students total $18 million in the form of a revolving loan fund; new loans are made only as old loans are paid back.

Most, but not all, loan programs are based on financial need and carry interest rates lower than those for commercial loans. These programs include Pell grants for undergraduate students of exceptional financial need, nursing student loans, national direct student loans, and guaranteed student loans. For the latter, students arrange for 8 percent loans through commercial lenders and the loans are backed by state or federal agencies.

Other sources of financial aid are drawn from the states and from the schools' own financial aid program. Each state has a different need-based financial aid program. Schools offer assistance, not necessarily based on financial need, that includes grants, loans, and work-study arrangements. Private and nonprofit organizations such as the NLN, the National Student Nurses' Association, and the American Cancer Society also sponsor scholarships for nursing students.

The availability of these funds is not nearly commensurate with need. Therefore, many students resort to part-time study in order to work while in school. For nurses employed by hospitals and other health agencies, tuition reimbursement is often available as a fringe benefit.

Q *What is the amount of federal support for nursing and nursing education? How does this compare with other health professions?*

A Federal support for nursing education, funded through the Division of Nursing in the form of grants to schools, student traineeships, and special projects, totaled approximately $58 million for fiscal year 1990. This compares with a total of $186 million in similar federal funding for other health professions.

In addition, federal spending for biomedical research at the National Institutes of Health totaled $8.3 billion. Of this money, $39 million is earmarked for nursing research grants funded through the National Center for Nursing Research. Under the Medicare program in fiscal year 1990, the medical profession received $980 million for graduate medical education, covering Medicare's share of interns' and residents' salaries. An additional $515 million covered the costs of nursing education, allied health professionals, classroom space, and other educational expenses to cover the higher costs of teaching hospitals.

Q *Why would a nurse obtain a PhD?*

A For similar reasons that one would obtain a PhD in other disciplines. A PhD prepares a nurse to conduct research and hence improve nursing practice. In addition, a PhD is often a minimum requirement for a teacher in a university or collegiate setting. As nurses strive to gain greater accountability for their practice and equal footing with colleagues in other areas of health care delivery, doctoral preparation is of increasing importance (Figure 4). Nurses with PhDs are needed as educators, as researchers of nursing practice, as administrators of nursing service, and as public policy experts who can make major contributions to health policy because of their familiarity with the clinical side of health care and their knowledge of policy analysis.

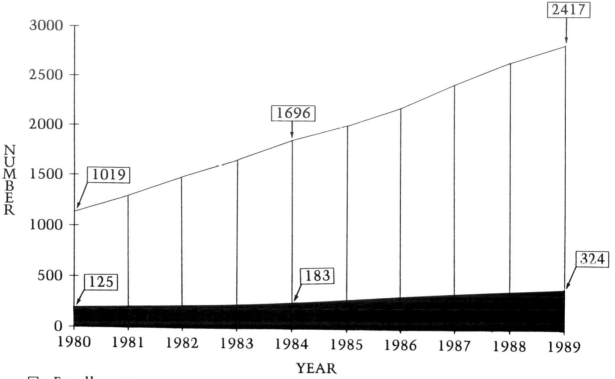

Figure 4. Enrollments and Graduations from Doctoral Programs in Nursing: 10-Year Trend

Q What is nursing research?

A Nursing research is scientific investigation that examines the biological, biomedical, and behavioral processes that underlie health and the environment in which health care is delivered. Most often research is conducted by graduate students, doctoral candidates, or faculty in schools of nursing. Also, many health care institutions now employ nurse researchers to conduct studies of particular relevance to their populations.

Researchable questions that are generated in practice might include the following: What methods can nurses use to prevent complications of hospitalizations, such as nosocomial infection, pressure necrosis, and thrombophlebitis? What teaching strategies, care modalities, and support interventions can decrease the length of stay of an oncology patient and permit an optimal life-style outside of the hospital?

When results of nursing care research are applied, patient care is improved. Better care costs less money in the long run. For example, Dr. Dorothy Brooten and her associates studied low birth weight, premature infants in intensive care units that were not discharged until they weighed 5 kilograms. The researchers found that if the infants were discharged earlier, they gained weight at home—and the family coped with the situation better. This information resulted in an average net savings of $18,560 per infant.

Fast Facts
About Nursing

Q *How many nurses are there in the United States?*

A As of March 1988, there were 2,033,032 registered nurses licensed to practice, an increase of about 45 percent since September 1977. Approximately 782,000 practical nurses are licensed to practice.

Q *How many men are there in nursing?*

A Approximately 67,000, or 3.3 percent, of all registered nurses are men.

Q *How many nurses are of minority ethnic background?*

A Approximately 75,000 (3.6 percent) are blacks; 47,000 (2.3 percent) are of Asian descent; 26,000 (1.3 percent) are Hispanic; and 8,000 (0.4 percent) are American Indians or Alaskan natives.

Q *How many men and minority students are enrolled in basic nursing programs?*

A For 1988, the approximate numbers and percentages of minority students enrolled in basic RN programs were as follows:

Type of Student	Number	Percentage
Men	10,100	6.2
Blacks	16,732	10.3
Hispanics	4,392	2.7
Asians	3,613	2.2
American Indians	876	0.5

Q *What percentage of nurses hold baccalaureate degrees?*

A Approximately 27 percent of the nurses in the nation have baccalaureate degrees. This percentage is increasing, as evidenced by NLN data that over 40,000 RNs enroll each year in baccalaureate nursing programs.

Q *What percentage of nurses hold master's degrees?*

A Approximately 5 percent of the RN population have master's degrees. The percentage will continue to rise; over 22,000 students now are enrolled in master's programs each year.

Q *What percentage of nurses hold doctoral degrees?*

A Fewer than 1 percent of the RNs in the nation hold doctoral degrees. This percentage is rising, as evidenced by yearly increases in the number of doctoral nursing programs (47 in 1989) and the subsequent increases in the numbers of nurses enrolled in those programs (2,417 in 1989).

Q *How many nursing schools are there?*

A There are 1,457 basic RN programs in the United States: 488 baccalaureate programs, 812 associate degree programs, and 157 diploma programs.

Q *How many nursing faculty members are there? What is their educational background?*

A There are approximately 16,813 full-time and 5,372 part-time nursing faculty members in the nation's RN programs. Approximately 74 percent of full-time faculty members have master's degrees, 19 percent have doctoral degrees, and 8 percent have baccalaureate degrees as their highest earned academic credential.

Q *How many national specialty organizations are there?*

A There are over 60 national specialty organizations. They meet twice a year as the National Federation of Nursing Specialty Organizations (NFNSO). NFNSO recently incorporated and has an elected executive committee comprised of a president, vice president, secretary, and treasurer. (See the listing of nursing organizations in the Resource List.)

Q *What is the function of the federal government's Division of Nursing?*

A The Division of Nursing is located within the Health Resources and Services Administration of the Public Health Service of the Department of Health and Human Services. Since the 1960s, it has been responsible for administering the federal government's funding of nursing education, both to nursing programs and individual nursing recipients. In 1990, the program's grants totaled $57.7 million.

Q *How many nurses hold federal or state offices?*

A According to the ANA political education department, 53 nurses have been elected as state representatives. Although no nurses have yet been elected to Congress, several have held key positions within the federal government. For example, from 1981 to 1985, Carolyne Davis, PhD, RN, was director of HCFA, the agency responsible for Medicare and Medicaid. Another nurse, O. Marie Henry, is the Deputy Surgeon General and Chief Nurse Officer for the Public Health Service. Sheila Burke, MPA, RN, FAAN, is chief of staff for Senate Minority Leader Robert Dole, and two nurses have served in the White House Office of Public Liaison.

Several other nurses have worked for legislators or congressional committees, have held prominent positions within the Department of Health and Human Services, or have been selected as White House fellows.

Q What is the function of The National Center for Nursing Research?

A The National Center for Nursing Research (NCNR), a part of the National Institutes of Health (NIH), was authorized under the Health Research Extension Act of 1985, P.L. 99-158. Although the President vetoed the bill, organized nursing collectively and successfully lobbied Congress who overwhelmingly overrode the veto, making the bill a law and the center a reality.

Under the direction of Ada Sue Hinshaw, PhD, RN, FAAN, the mission of the NCNR is "the conduct and support of, and dissemination of information respecting, basic and clinical nursing research, training, and other programs in patient care research." The research programs of the NCNR address actual and potential health problems. These programs focus on health promotion, mitigation of the effects of acute and chronic illnesses and disabilities, and delivery of nursing services.

The center was originally proposed by Representative Edward Madigan (R-Illinois), with the intent to transfer to the center the research activities previously conducted at the Division of Nursing and place nursing research more in the mainstream of the federal government's health care research activities. Its funding for fiscal year 1990 totaled $39 million.

Resource List

Statistical Sources

American Nurses' Association. (1987). *Facts about Nursing '86–87*. Kansas City, MO: Author.

American Nurses' Association. (1990). *The Nursing Shortage and the 1990s: Realities and Remedies*. Kansas City, MO: Author.

National League for Nursing. (1991). *Licensed to Care: An Executive Report on the New Nurse*. New York: National League for Nursing.

National League for Nursing. (1989). *Nurse Faculty: Socioeconomic Trends*. New York: National League for Nursing.

National League for Nursing. (1990). *Nursing Data Review 1989*. New York: National League for Nursing.

National League for Nursing. (1990). *Nursing DataSource 1990: A Research Bulletin with Public Policy Briefs*. New York: National League for Nursing.

National League for Nursing. (1989). *Nursing Student Census with Policy Implications 1989*. New York: National League for Nursing.

National League for Nursing. (1989). *Profiles of the Newly Licensed Nurse*. New York: National League for Nursing.

National League for Nursing. (1990). *State-Approved Schools of Nursing LPN/LVN-1990*. New York: National League for Nursing.

National League for Nursing. (1990). *State-Approved Schools of Nursing RN-1990*. New York: National League for Nursing.

U.S. Department of Health and Human Services. (1988). *The Registered Nurse Population, 1988*. Washington, DC: Author.

U.S. Department of Health and Human Services. (1988). *Seventh Report to the President and Congress on the Status of Health Personnel in the United States*. Washington, DC: Bureau of the Health Professions, Health Resources and Services Administration, Department of Health and Human Services.

Annotated Bibliography

American Medical Association Center for Health Services Research. (1978, January). The nurse practitioner role in the delivery setting. *Journal of the American Medical Association, 330,* 486–490.

Nurse practitioners deliver care at a considerable cost savings.

American Nurses' Association and the National Association of Pediatric Nurse Associates and Practitioners. (1984, February). Nurse practitioners: A review of the research. *Nursing Outlook, 32*(1), 84.

Review of nearly 30 studies evidencing the favorable impact of the nurse practitioner on quality and type of care delivered. Findings include:

- Nurse practitioners achieve better control of obesity and hypertension in their patients when compared with physicians.
- Eighty-six percent of nurse practitioners' patients gained satisfactory relief from symptoms compared with 73 percent of the physicians' patients. NPs were found to identify signs and symptoms and possess greater knowledge of the patient's problems.
- Patients of nurse practitioners were found to visit emergency rooms or other physicians less frequently.
- Hospitalization and length of stay were markedly reduced among chronically ill elderly persons in homes and nursing homes using nurse practitioners with physician consultation.

Amado, A., et al. (1979, August). Cost of terminal care: Home hospice v. hospital. *Nursing Outlook, 27,* 522–526.

Demonstration project to determine if an intensive array of fully reimbursed home services would reduce the dying patient's use of hospital days of care. The total cost of care for all patients in the study was $118,626 for 1,576 days of care. Physicians estimated that 943 hospital days of care would otherwise have been required, at an approximate cost of $212,175.

Brooten, D., et al. (1986, October). A randomized clinical trial of early hospital discharge and home follow-up of very-low-birth-weight infants. *New England Journal of Medicine, 315,* 934–939.

Study compared nursing services in the home with hospitalization for the care of very-low-birth-weight infants and found considerable cost savings, with no lowering of quality outcomes, for nurse-managed home care. Net savings was calculated at $18,560 per infant, or 25.6 percent of charges for control (hospitalized) group.

Burnip, R., et al. (1976, January). Well-child care by pediatric nurse practitioners in a large group practice. *American Journal of Dis. Child, 130,* 51–55.

Pediatric nurse practitioners shown to be competent, productive, accepted, and cost-effective compared with physicians.

Caward, J. (1981, November-December). Economics of the nurse practitioner role in an industrial setting. *Nurse Practitioner, 6,* 17.

When a newly trained nurse practitioner was added to a small industrial company's health service, the company estimated its savings on "industrials, medicals, taxi transportation, and lost work time to be . . . a mean savings of $3,621 a month."

Civilian Health and Medical Program of the Uniformed Services (CHAMPUS). (1980). *Reimbursement to nurse practitioners.* Washington, DC: Author.

Study conducted to determine cost-effectiveness of direct, independent reimbursement to NPs. In 75 percent of the providers' billings studied, cost was 31 percent less than the limit allowed for physicians.

Colt, A. M., et al. (1977, October). Home health care is good economics. *Nursing Outlook, 25,* 632–636.

Demonstration project of the Metropolitan Nursing Health Services Association of Rhode Island examined the demand for maintenance services and cost-effectiveness among patients who had exhausted their Medicare coverage for home visits or who needed, but were not financially eligible for, home health aide services through welfare funding. The home maintenance program helped save Medicare or state medical assistance programs $855 per enrollee per year, equaling $85,000 for every hundred patients.

Cunningham, N., et al. (1978, December). Telemedicine: Favorable experience in pediatric primary care. *Journal of the American Medical Association, 204,* 2749–2751.

Demonstrated that nurse practitioners had slightly more effective communications with patients than physician counterparts.

Fagin, C. M. (1982, January). Nursing as an alternative to high-cost care. *American Journal of Nursing, 82,* 56–60.

Overview of literature indicating that nurses provide many primary care services as well as, and less expensively than, physicians.

Friedman, J. (1987, June). Hospital care comes home: Home health staffers give high-tech, high-touch care—some even do windows. *American Health, 17,* 18.

Travenol, a national firm providing high-tech equipment and home services at prices below hospital charges, estimates dialysis costs $14,500 per year at home, compared with $23,000 at a clinic. Home chemotherapy costs $42,500 versus $126,000 in a hospital. Total parental nutrition costs $73,000 at home versus $200,000 in the hospital.

Hammond, J. (1979, July-August). Home health care cost-effectiveness: An overview of the literature. *Public Health Report, 94,* 305–311.

Literature review yielded the following conclusions:

- Home care is less expensive than institutionalization from the standpoint of third-party underwriters.
- Available studies indicate that home health care has a potential for averting the hospitalization of some patients.
- Early discharge with subsequent home health care generally reduces the cost per case to the underwriter.
- The costs of extended care services, whether provided in the institution or in the home, are roughly equivalent.

Hegyvary, S., et al. (1988, February). Research on strategies for maintaining quality in the delivery of patient care. Panel

Presentation: *Nursing Resources and the Delivery of Patient Care*, Invitational Conference, National Center for Nursing Research, U.S. Department of Health and Human Services/ NIH, pp. 19–20.

Summary of existing research concluded:

- Competency of nurses and good nurse/physician communication contribute more to a decreased mortality rate in intensive care units than the presence of high technologies.
- Some specific nursing interventions are cost-effective, although most nursing interventions have not been studied for their cost-effectiveness.
- Nurse practitioners, certified nurse-midwives, and physicians' assistants provide high quality care at reduced costs with the cost savings passed on to consumers and third-party payers.
- Additional factors have been shown to relate to quality of care, including early discharge and home nursing for low-birth-weight infants, and the quality of temporary agency nurses.

Jones, K. (1975, December). Study documents effect of primary nursing on renal transplant patients. *Hospitals, 49,* 85–89.

Study conducted at the University of Michigan Medical Center in Ann Arbor demonstrating the effectiveness of the clinical nurse specialist in caring for renal transplant patients. Conclusions showed an average reduction of three weeks in hospital stay and significantly fewer complications suffered by the patients receiving primary nursing. Actual savings for this very small group of patients was more than $51,000.

Lubic, R. (1980). Evaluation of an out-of-hospital maternity center for low-risk patients. In L. H. Aiken (Ed.), *Health Policy and Nursing Practice* (pp. 90–116). New York: McGraw-Hill Book Co.

In outpatient care, nurse practitioners were shown to provide many primary care services with a higher degree of patient satisfaction at a lower cost than physicians.

Martinson, I. M., et al. (1978, February). Facilitating home care for children dying of cancer. *Cancer Nursing, 1,* 41–45.

Martinson, I. M., et al. (1978, July). Home care for children dying of cancer. *Pediatrics, 62,* 106–113.

Studies found that hospital care was approximately 18 times more expensive then was the cost of home care. The mean cost of home care was $827 per child, with an average cost per day of $25. Comparable rates for hospital care were $200 per day, with a mean cost of $13,022.

McCarthy, C. (1975, December). Incentive reimbursement as an impetus to cost containment. *Inquiry, 12*, 320–329.

The Social Security Administration, experimenting with financial incentives to reduce costs, financed a project of the Health Insurance Plan of Greater New York in which one nurse was assigned to each of six medical groups. The nurses' patient populations included Medicare recipients suffering from chronic conditions that were likely to entail frequent physician visits and possible hospitalizations. "Assessment of the first year of program operation showed a decline both in hospitalization and in length of stay that was greater among HIP Medicare patients than among the control group."

Miller, F. N. (1985, January-February). Nurse providers: A resource for growing population needs. *Business and Health*, 38–42.

Ninety-five percent of all health care resources are spent on 5 percent of the problem. That 5 percent represents the medical care needed to pull a patient through an acute illness. Little is spent on health care to keep a person in a state of wellness.

Miller, M. K., & Stokes, C. S. (1978, September). Health status, health resources, and consolidated structural parameters: Implications for public health care policy. *Journal of Health and Social Behavior, 19*, 263–279.

Nationwide study of the relative impacts of health care services resources and community structure on two measures of physical health status—infant mortality and age-sex adjusted death rates. The only health resource that made an apparent difference in positive outcome was the increase in nurses per capita.

Muller, C., et al. (1977, March). Cost factors in urban telemedicine. *Medical Care, 15*, 251–259.

Evidence that nurse practitioners alter the delivery of medical services in a way that improves access and reduces costs.

Noelker, L., & Harel, Z. (1978, February). Aged excluded from home health care: An interorganizational solution. *Gerontologist, 18*, 37–41.

Study conducted by the Visiting Nurse Association (VNA) and two other Cleveland organizations. A cooperative home extension program for elderly people who were not eligible for Medicare and home health benefits was established. After one year only 13 percent of the Chronic Illness Center's clients and none of the VNA clients required institutionalization.

Prescott, P. A., & Sorensen, J. F. (1978, fall). Cost-effectiveness analysis: An approach to evaluating nursing programs. *Nursing Administration, 3*, 17–40.

Analysis of literature on cost-effectiveness of nursing, and model for documenting cost-effectiveness.

Ross, M. G. (1981, November-December). Health impact of a nurse-midwife program. *Nursing Research, 30*, 353–355.

Study of nurse-midwifery services provided to the Navaho Indian population at Fort Defiance, Arizona. Major findings:

- A significant association between increased prenatal care and a decreased percentage of hospitalized infants.
- The average maternal hospital stay for labor and delivery was lessened by an average of three-fourths of a day.
- Fewer forceps deliveries and cesarean sections were noted in the population served by the midwives.
- Lower incidence of prematurity observed among the patients treated by midwives.
- Significant reduction in infant morbidity in the community served by the nurse-midwifery program.

Runyan, J. W., Jr. (1975, January). The Memphis chronic disease program: Comparisons in outcome and the nurses' extended role. *Journal of the American Medical Association, 231*, 264–267.

Control group receiving physician services was compared with an experimental group receiving services from nurse practitioners. Those in the nurse practitioner group were found to have lower blood pressures, lower blood sugars, and fewer hospitalizations.

Schultz, P. R., & McGlone, F. B. (1977, October). Primary health care provided to the elderly by a nurse practitioner/physician team: Analysis of cost-effectiveness. *Journal of the American Geriatric Society, 25*, 443–446.

Study compared two staffing methods in delivery of primary care: physician only (PO) and adult health nurse practitioner/physician (NP/P) team. Concluded that NP/P team was substantially more cost-efficient (almost 50 percent less costly) in its system of health care delivery for home-bound patients.

Swenson, J. P. (1981, October). Training patients to administer intravenous antibiotics at home. *American Journal of Hospital Pharmacology, 38*, 1480–1483.

Substantial savings in hospitalization time and treatment expense was noted through the home intravenous antibiotic program. Savings averaged 16 hospital days and $2,371 per patient.

Weissart, W. G. (1978, March). Costs of adult day care: Comparison to nursing homes. *Inquiry, 15*, 10–19.

Weissart, W. G. (1979, winter). Rationales for public health insurance coverage of geriatric day care: Issues, options, and impacts. *Journal of Health Policy Law, 3*, 555–567.

Weissart, W. G., et al. (1980, June). Effects and costs of day care services for the chronically ill: A randomized experiment. *Medical Care, 18*, 567–584.

Weissart's studies demonstrated that the cost of adult day care in comparison to nursing homes could result in a potential savings of 37 to 60 percent of the cost of nursing home care, depending on frequency of day care center use.

Widmer, G., et al. (1978, August). Home health care services and cost. *Nursing Outlook, 26*, 488–493.

Study of home health care by a visiting nurse association of New York and the New York City Health Systems Agency. The median cost per patient in the study was $347 compared to $1,280 per month in a skilled nursing facility.

Health Policy Journals
and Newsletters

American Journal of Public Health
American Public Health Association
1015 15th Street, NW
Washington, DC 20005

Business and Health
Washington Business Group on Health
229-1/2 Pennsylvania Avenue, SE
Washington, DC 20003

Capital Update
American Nurses' Association
1101 14th Street, NW
Washington, DC 20005

Health Affairs
Project HOPE
Millwood, VA 22646

Health Policy Week
United Communications Group
4550 Montgomery Avenue, #700 N.
Bethesda, MD 20814

Home Health Line
Karen Rak Publisher
Port Republic, MD 20676

Hospitals
American Hospital Publishing, Inc.
211 East Chicago Avenue
Chicago, IL 60611

*Inquiry: The Journal of Health Care Organization, Provision,
and Finance*
Blue Cross Blue Shield Association
P.O. Box 527
Glenview, IL 60025

Journal of Health Politics, Policy and Law
Duke University Press
T. R. Marnor, Department of Health Administration
Corner of Erwin Road and Trent Drive
Duke University
Durham, NC 27710

Legislative Network for Nurses
Legislative Network for Nurses, Inc.
P.O. Box 40071
L'Enfant Plaza, SW
Washington, DC 20026

Medical Benefits
Kelley Communications
410 East Water Street
Charlottesville, VA 22901

Modern Healthcare
Crain Communications
740 Rush Street
Chicago, IL 60611

Nursing and Health Care
National League for Nursing
350 Hudson Street
New York, NY 10014

Washington Actions on Health
Capitol Publications
1101 King Street
Alexandria, VA 22313

Books on Political Science, Policy, and Government

Aiken, L. (Ed.). (1981). *Health policy and nursing practice.* New York: McGraw-Hill.

Aiken, L., & Gortner, S. (Eds.). (1982). *Nursing in the 1980s: Crises, opportunities, challenges.* Philadelphia: J.B. Lippincott.

American Nurses' Association. (1980). *Nursing: A social policy statement.* Kansas City: Author.

Bagwell, M., & Clements, S. (1985). *A political handbook for health professionals.* Boston: Little, Brown.

Califano, J. A., Jr. (1986). *America's health care revolution: Who lives? who dies? who pays?* New York: Random House.

Dahl, R. (1976). *Modern political analysis.* Englewood Cliffs, NJ: Prentice-Hall.

Government Printing Office. Congressional Record, Federal Register, Digest of Public General Bills and Resolutions. Washington, DC: Author.

Institute of Medicine. (1983). *Nursing and nursing education: Public policies and private actions.* Washington, DC: National Academy Press.

Kalisch, B. J., & Kalisch, P. A. (1982). *Politics of nursing.* Philadelphia: J.B. Lippincott.

Lasswell, R. (1958). *Politics: Who gets what, when, how.* New York: Peter Smith.

Mason, D., & Talbott, S. (1985). *Political action handbook for nurses.* Menlo Park, CA: Addison-Wesley.

Redman, E. (1973). *The dance of the legislation.* New York: Simon and Schuster.

Solomon, S. B., & Roe, S. C. (1986). *Integrating health policy into the curriculum.* New York: National League for Nursing.

Solomon, S. B., & Roe, S. C. (1986). *Key concepts in public policy: Student workbook.* New York: National League for Nursing.

Stevens, K. R. (Ed.). (1983). *Power and influence: A source book for nurses.* New York: John Wiley & Sons.

Verba, F., & Nie, N. H. (1972). *Participation in America: Political democracy and social equality.* New York: Harper & Row.

Nursing Organizations

American Nurses' Association
2420 Pershing Road
Kansas City, MO 64108
Tel. (816) 474-5720

American Academy of Ambulatory Nursing Administration
N. Woodbury Road, Box 56
Pitman, NJ 08071
Tel. (609) 582-9617

American Academy of Nurse Practitioners
45 Foster Street, Suite A
Lowell, MA 01851
Tel. (512) 442-4262

The American Assembly for Men in Nursing
P.O. Box 31753
Independence, OH 44131

American Association of Colleges of Nursing
One Dupont Circle, NW, Suite 530
Washington, DC 20036
Tel. (202) 463-6930

American Association of Critical-Care Nurses
One Civic Plaza, Suite 330
Newport Beach, CA 92660
Tel. (714) 644-9310

American Association of Neuroscience Nurses
218 N. Jefferson, Suite 204
Chicago, IL 60606
Tel. (312) 993-0043

American Association of Nurse Anesthetists
216 Higgins Road
Park Ridge, IL 60068
Tel. (312) 692-7050

American Association of Occupational Health Nurses, Inc.
50 Lenox Pointe
Atlanta, GA 30324
Tel. (404) 262-1162

American College of Nurse-Midwives
1522 K Street, NW, Suite 1000
Washington, DC 20005
Tel. (202) 289-0171

American Holistic Nurses' Association
4101 Lake Boon Drive, Suite 201
Raleigh, NC 27607
Tel. (919) 787-0116

American Hospital Association
840 N. Lake Shore Drive
Chicago, IL 60611
Tel. (312) 280-6000

American Nephrology Nurses' Association
N. Woodbury Road, Box 56
Pitman, NJ 08071
Tel. (609) 589-2187

American Organization of Nurse Executives
840 N. Lake Shore Drive, 10E
Chicago, IL 60611
Tel. (312) 280-5213

American Society of Ophthalmic Registered Nurses, Inc.
P.O. Box 193030
San Francisco, CA 94119
Tel. (415) 561-8513

American Society of Plastic & Reconstructive Surgical
Nurses, Inc.
N. Woodbury Road, Box 56
Pitman, NJ 08071
Tel. (609) 589-6247

American Society of Post Anesthesia Nurses
11512 Allecingie Parkway
Richmond, VA 23235
Tel. (804) 379-5516

American Urological Association Allied, Inc.
11512 Allecingie Parkway
Richmond, VA 23235

Association for the Care of Children's Health
3615 Wisconsin Avenue, NW
Washington, DC 20016
Tel. (202) 244-1801

Association of Operating Room Nurses
10170 E. Mississippi Avenue
Denver, CO 80231
Tel. (303) 755-6300

Association of Pediatric Oncology Nurses
11512 Allecingie Parkway
Richmond, VA 23235
Tel. (804) 379-1386

Association for Practitioners in Infection Control
505 E. Hawley Street
Mundelein, IL 60060
Tel. (312) 949-6052

Association of Rehabilitation Nurses
5700 Old Orchard Road, 1st floor
Skokie, IL 60077
Tel. (708) 966-3433

Dermatology Nurses Association
N. Woodbury Road, Box 56
Pitman, NJ 08071
Tel. (609) 582-1915

Emergency Nurses Association
230 East Ohio, 6th floor
Chicago, IL 60611
Tel. (312) 649-0297

International Association for Enterostomal Therapy, Inc.
2081 Business Center Drive, Suite 290
Irvine, CA 92715
Tel. (714) 476-0268

Intravenous Nurses Society, Inc.
Two Brighton Street
Belmont, MA 02178
Tel. (617) 489-5205

Lesbian and Gay Nurses Alliance
801 E. Harrison, Suite 106
Seattle, WA 98102

National Alliance of Nurse Practitioners
P.O. Box 44707
L'Enfant Plaza, SW
Washington, DC 20026

National Association for Health Care Recruitment
P.O. Box 5769
Akron, OH 44372
Tel. (216) 867-3088

National Association of Hispanic Nurses
2300 W. Commerce Street, Suite 300
San Antonio, TX 78207
Tel. (512) 226-9743

National Association of Orthopaedic Nurses, Inc.
N. Woodbury Road, P.O. Box 56
Pitman, NJ 08071
Tel. (609) 582-0111

National Association of Pediatric Nurse Associates and
Practitioners
1101 Kings Highway, Suite 206
Cherry Hill, NJ 08034
Tel. (609) 667-7773

National Association of School Nurses, Inc.
Lamplighter Lane, P.O. Box 1300
Scarborough, ME 04074
Tel. (207) 883-2117

National Flight Nurses Association
P.O. Box 371365
San Diego, CA 92137-1365
Tel. (619) 223-2746

National League for Nursing
350 Hudson Street
New York, NY 10014
Tel. (212) 989-9393

National Nurses Society on Addictions
5700 Old Orchard Road, 1st floor
Skokie, IL 60077
Tel. (708) 966-5010

Nurses Association of the American College of Obstetricians
and Gynecologists
409 12th Street, SW
Washington, DC 20024
Tel. (202) 863-2439

Nurse Consultants Association, Inc.
414 Plaza Drive, Suite 209
Westmont, IL 60559
Tel. (312) 655-0087

Nurses Organization of the Veterans Administration
6728 Old McLean Village Drive
McLean, Virginia 22101
Tel. (703) 556-9222

Oncology Nursing Society
1016 Greentree Road
Pittsburgh, PA 15220-3125
Tel. (412) 921-7373

Public Health Nursing/American Public Health Association
1015 Fifteenth Street, NW
Washington, DC 20005
Tel. (202) 789-5600

Society of Gastrointestinal Assistants, Inc.
1070 Sibley Tower
Rochester, NY 14604
Tel. (716) 546-7241

Society for Peripheral Vascular Nursing
309 Winter Street
Norwood, MA 02062
Tel. (617) 762-3630

Society of Otorhinolaryngology and Head-Neck Nurses, Inc.
439 N. Causeway
New Smyrna Beach, FL 32169
Tel. (904) 428-1695

Frequently Used Abbreviations

American Association of Colleges of Nursing (AACN)

American Association of Retired Persons (AARP)

American Medical Association (AMA)

American Nurses' Association (ANA)

American Organization of Nurse Executives (AONE)

Community Health Accreditation Program (CHAP)

Certified Nurse-Midwife (CNM)

Community Nursing Organization (CNO)

Certified Registered Nurse Anesthetist (CRNA)

Diagnostic Related Groups (DRGs)

Health Care Financing Administration (HCFA)

Health Maintenance Organization (HMO)

Institute of Medicine (IOM)

National Center for Nursing Research (NCNR)

National Federation of Nursing Specialty Organizations (NFNSO)

National Institutes of Health (NIH)

National League for Nursing (NLN)

Nurse Practitioner (NP)

Physician Payment Review Commission (PPRC)

Political Action Committee (PAC)

Preferred Provider Organizations (PPO)

Prospective Payment Review Commission (PROPAC)

Prospective Payment System (PPS)

Public Service Announcement (PSA)

Resource-Based Relative Value Scale (RBRVS)

Registered Care Technologist (RCT)